Management of Type 1 Diabetes

First Edition

Irl B. Hirsch, MD

Professor of Medicine
University of Washington, Seattle

Steven V. Edelman, MD

Professor of Medicine
Division of Endocrinology and Metabolism
University of California, San Diego
Veterans Affairs Medical Center

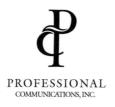

PROFESSIONAL
COMMUNICATIONS, INC.

Professional Communications, Inc.

A Medical Publishing Company

Marketing Office:
400 Center Bay Drive
West Islip, NY 11795
(t) 631/661-2852
(f) 631/661-2167

Editorial Office:
PO Box 10
Caddo, OK 74729-0010
(t) 580/367-9838
(f) 580/367-9989

For orders only, please call
1-800-337-9838

or visit our website at
www.pcibooks.com

ISBN: 1-884735-94-0

Printed in the United States of America

DISCLAIMER

This text is printed on recycled paper.

DEDICATION

ACKNOWLEDGMENT

We gratefully acknowledge the editorial assistance of Carol Verderese in the preparation of the book.

TABLE OF CONTENTS

TABLES

FIGURES

The authors know about type 1 diabetes all too well, as we both have lived with this condition for about 70 years combined. We have seen tremendous progress in the tools for treatment, with the development of home glucose monitors, fast- and long-acting insulin analogues, insulin pumps and pens, and diabetes management software programs. Both of us can recall when the only home monitoring option was the burdensome and unhelpful urine test, and there was little to do for the high urine sugars since once- or twice-daily insulin was the rule. Indeed, the impurity of those older products often caused skin problems, a side effect that is virtually unheard of today. Still, despite these major diagnostic and therapeutic advances, diabetes care remains inadequate and poorly understood in the majority of individuals living with this largely self-managed autoimmune disease.

A person with type 1 diabetes must be aware of their condition every minute of every day and night. The common phrase "24/7" captures life with type 1 diabetes quite well. During the day, there is a constant struggle to prevent and treat wide, unexpected, and extremely frustrating fluctuations in glucose levels while trying to conduct a normal life. At nighttime, it seems like a crap shoot whether your regimen will lead to a sweat-drenched, nightmare-ridden hypoglycemic reaction or a revolving door to the toilet and water faucet, trying to slake an unquenchable thirst due to hyperglycemia. It is virtually impossible to fully appreciate the challenges without living it yourself, or with your spouse or child.

This is one of the first books specifically addressing type 1 diabetes in adults written by two individuals who not only have lived with this condition a long time, but have dedicated their careers to caring for people afflicted with this demanding disease.

1　Epidemiology

Type 1 diabetes is a chronic disease resulting from the autoimmune destruction of insulin-producing pancreatic β cells. Slightly more than 218,000 cases of type 1 diabetes are diagnosed annually worldwide and approximately 40% of these newly diagnosed patients are children under 15 years of age. Type 1 diabetes is the third most common serious chronic disease of childhood after asthma and mental retardation. It is associated with severe morbidity and mortality when not properly treated and places a prodigious burden on health care resources, making it a prime target for prevention.

According to the International Diabetes Federation (IDF), the incidence of type 1 diabetes is greatest among people of northern European descent, with approximately 60,000 new cases reported annually. The incidence is highest in Finland and has been rising: in 1953, the rate of diagnosis of new patients with type 1 diabetes <15 years of age was 12/100,000 vs 36/100,000 during the years 1987 to 1990. Southeast Asia has the second-highest annual incidence (~45,000), followed by North America (~36,000). Of the IDF regions, Africa has the lowest number of new cases annually (~6,900), but the proportion of children is highest there, at approximately 54% (**Figure 1.1**). In the United States, the annual incidence was 12 to 14 per 100,000 during the 1990s, increasing from an almost complete absence in early infancy to peak onset around the years of puberty.

The prevalence of type 1 diabetes worldwide is approximately 5.3 million, and about 7.4% of these cases are children ≤14 years of age. The largest popu-

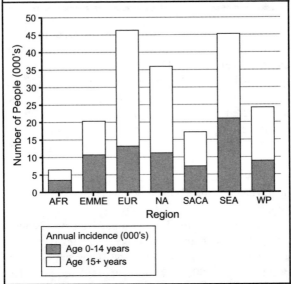

FIGURE 1.1 — Estimated Incidence of Type 1 Diabetes by International Diabetes Federation Region

Abbreviations: AFR, Africa; EMME, Eastern Mediterranian and Middle East; EUR, Europe; NA, North America; SACA, South and Central America; SEA, Southeast Asia; WP, Western Pacific.

From: http://www.eatlas.idf.org.

lation is found in Europe (~1.6 million), followed by North America (~1 million), and Southeast Asia (~920,000). Scandinavia has the highest prevalence rates, while China and Japan have the lowest. During the 1990s, the prevalence of type 1 diabetes in the United States in people <20 years of age was about 0.26% and the lifetime prevalence nearly 0.4%. This translates into approximately 1 million Americans with type 1 diabetes.

Regional variations in the development of type 1 diabetes are attributed to the frequency of high-risk HLA alleles in racially distinct populations. However, diet and environmental factors may also play a role. For example, a higher incidence of the disease has been observed among children who were not breast-fed or were breast-fed only briefly, and increasing incidence in certain European countries is thought to result from environmental influences. These hypotheses are further supported by the findings that the disease develops in only 33% of the identical twins of study subjects and that 90% of patients with newly diagnosed type 1 diabetes do not have an affected first-degree relative.

Improvements in the ability to identify individuals at high risk for type 1 diabetes, together with encouraging results of interventions in animal models, have provided the impetus for large multicenter clinical trials focused on disease prevention. While results have been disappointing so far, it is widely believed that successful prevention will depend on initiating therapy early in the natural history of this disease. Deeper understanding of the pathogenesis of type 1 diabetes is likely to expand options for prevention and treatment and reverse epidemiologic portents of the rising toll of this disease throughout the world.

SUGGESTED READING

Atkinson MA, Maclaren NK. The pathogenesis of insulin-dependent diabetes mellitus. *N Engl J Med*. 1994;331:1428-1436.

International Diabetes Federation. E-Atlas. http://www.eatlas.idf.org. Accessed March 30, 2005.

Rewers M, LaPorte RE, King H, Tuomilehto J. Trends in the prevalence and incidence of diabetes: insulin-dependent diabetes mellitus in childhood. *World Health Stat Q*. 1988;41:179-189.

Tuomilehto J, Karvonen M, Pitkäniemi J, et al. Record-high incidence of type 1 (insulin-dependent) diabetes mellitus in Finnish children. The Finnish Childhood Type 1 Diabetes Registry Group. *Diabetologia.* 1999;42:655-660.

2 Mechanisms of Fuel Metabolism

Optimal diabetes management consists of manipulating or adjusting the mechanisms of fuel metabolism to approximate normal physiology as closely as possible. Although complete normalization of fuel metabolism remains an elusive goal, increased understanding of the multihormonal components of glucose homeostasis, described below, has led to intensive therapeutic strategies that can yield near-normal glycemic control in patients with diabetes.

Normal Fuel Metabolism

Fuel metabolism is regulated by the complex interplay of:
- Multiple tissues and organs
- Intracellular enzymatic systems
- Hormones and other factors that mediate:
  - Distribution of ingested nutrients to organs and tissues
  - Storage of excess nutrients as glycogen or fat
  - Release of energy from storage depots to accommodate fasting or high-energy output.

■ Carbohydrate Metabolism

Carbohydrate in the form of glucose is a prime source of energy for muscles and the brain. The two main sources of circulating glucose are hepatic glucose production and ingested carbohydrate. During fasting, the glucoregulatory hormone glucagon stimulates the liver to produce plasma glucose through the processes of glycogenolysis and gluconeogenesis. This

17

is referred to as basal glucose production, and it is essential to preventing hypoglycemia and supplying sufficient amounts of glucose to the brain.

Ingested carbohydrate is hydrolyzed into component sugars during gut absorption, causing a postprandial rise in blood glucose level that reaches its peak 90 to 120 minutes after eating. The degree and rate of blood glucose elevation are determined by several factors, including the amount of carbohydrate ingested, the physical form of the food (eg, solid or liquid), and the amount and effect of insulin. The level of the neuroendocrine hormone amylin, which is cosecreted with insulin (**Figure 2.1**), also plays a key role in modulating postprandial glucose levels by suppressing postprandial glucagon production and regulating the rate of gastric emptying. As much as 70% of the oral carbohydrate load is stored as glycogen or fat (mostly glycogen), while the remainder is oxidized to meet immediate energy needs.

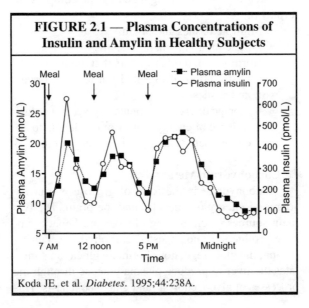

FIGURE 2.1 — Plasma Concentrations of Insulin and Amylin in Healthy Subjects

Koda JE, et al. *Diabetes*. 1995;44:238A.

■ Protein Metabolism

Ingested protein, absorbed as amino acids, is used for:

- Synthesis of new protein
- Oxidation to produce energy
- Conversion to glucose (gluconeogenesis).

During fasting, conversion of protein to glucose is essential to maintaining adequate glycemic levels.

■ Fat Metabolism

Fat is stored as triglyceride and converted to free fatty acids plus glycerol by lipolysis. Much of the ingested fat in a meal is stored in adipose tissue or muscle fat deposits. Free fatty acids from adipose tissue may be transported to the muscle for oxidation, which in turn produces ketone bodies that may be further metabolized as a source of energy. Chronic nutritional excess results in the accumulation of stored fat synthesized by excess glucose. Elevated circulating free fatty acids from ingested fat or lipolysis may inhibit peripheral insulin effect, slow the postabsorptive decline in blood glucose, and increase endothelial dysfunction.

Glucoregulatory Hormones

Fuel metabolism is regulated by numerous hormones acting in concert with the central nervous system. The extent and nature of these mechanisms are not fully understood. The key glucoregulatory hormones and their effects are described below.

■ Insulin

Insulin acts by increasing glucose uptake for oxidation and storage and by decreasing glucose production. The two forms of insulin secretion are basal and postprandial. Basal secretion produces relatively constant, low insulin levels that restrain lipolysis and the production of glucose. Abnormally low basal insulin secretion during fasting can cause hyperglycemia, hyperlipidemia, and ketosis. Insulin secretion also declines during exercise when glucose production and lipolysis are required to make stored energy available to tissues. β cells of the pancreatic islet are responsible for coordinating insulin secretion to changes in glycemia. Postprandial insulin secretion rises rapidly to accommodate higher blood glucose levels associated with nutrient intake. Elevated postprandial insulin levels suspend glucose production and lipolysis and stimulate uptake of ingested glucose by tissues.

■ Glucagon

Glucagon rises rapidly to stimulate hepatic glucose production when blood glucose levels fall, thereby preventing hypoglycemia in healthy individuals. In people with type 1 diabetes, glucagon secretion in response to hypoglycemia is absent after 3 to 5 years for reasons that are not yet understood. Furthermore, with eating, there is a paradoxical increase in glucagon levels. Therefore, in insulin-deficient patients, not only is insulin secretion inadequate to dispose of glucose peripherally, glucagon secretion is uncontrolled, leading to an increase in hepatic glucose output.

■ Amylin

Amylin is cosecreted with insulin to regulate glucose levels in the bloodstream. It complements the action of insulin by suppressing postprandial glucagon, which in turn decreases hepatic glucose production. Amylin also suppresses postprandial triglyceride concentrations and has been shown to reduce markers of oxidative stress and endothelial dysfunction. Additionally, it regulates gastric emptying that controls the rate of nutrient delivery into the circulation. People with diabetes have a deficiency in the secretion of amylin that matches the deficiency of insulin secretion, resulting in an excessive inflow of glucose into the bloodstream following meals.

■ Catecholamines

Catecholamines stimulate the release of stored energy during times of stress. They are the primary protection against hypoglycemia in patients with type 1 diabetes who have lost their glucagon response to hypoglycemia. Hypoglycemia unawareness and delayed recovery from hypoglycemia may occur when this defense is impaired.

■ Cortisol

Another "stress hormone," cortisol stimulates gluconeogenesis. However, it is less efficient than glucagon in this regard and thus is not as effective in protecting against acute hypoglycemia.

■ Growth Hormone

A surge of growth hormone secretion occurs during sleep, prompting a rise in blood glucose levels in the early morning referred to as the "dawn phenomenon." In individuals with normal metabolism, a slight increase in insulin secretion offsets the effects of growth hormone. However, in people with diabetes, variable nocturnal secretion of growth hormone often results in morning hyperglycemia.

SUGGESTED READING

Johnson LR, ed. *Essential Medical Physiology*. 2nd ed. Philadelphia, Pa: Lippincott-Raven; 1998.

Klingensmith GJ, ed. *Intensive Diabetes Management*. 3rd ed. Alexandria, Va: American Diabetes Association; 2003.

Levetan C, Want LL, Weyer C, et al. Impact of pramlintide on glucose fluctuations and postprandial glucose, glucagon, and triglyceride excursions among patients with type 1 diabetes intensively treated with insulin pumps. *Diabetes Care*. 2003;26:1-8.

Unger RH, Foster DW. Diabetes mellitus. In: Wilson JD, Foster DW, eds. *Williams Textbook of Endocrinology*. 8th ed. Philadelphia, Pa: WB Saunders Co; 1992:1273-1275.

3   Classification

Diabetes mellitus is a heterogeneous disease characterized metabolically by hyperglycemia and altered glucose metabolism. Historically, the disease was classified as either type 1, referred to as insulin-dependent diabetes mellitus (IDDM) or juvenile-onset diabetes, or type 2, commonly called non–insulin-dependent diabetes mellitus (NIDDM) or adult-onset diabetes. The American Diabetes Association (ADA) has recently revised this classification system, moving away from a framework based largely on the type of pharmacologic treatment used to one that is derived from current understanding of the etiology of the disease (**Table 3**.1).

Type 1 diabetes is divided into type 1A and type 1B, both of which feature severe insulin deficiency that leads to dependency on exogenous insulin therapy for survival. Type 1A diabetes is immune-mediated and defined by the presence of anti-islet autoantibodies, whereas type 1B is "idiopathic" insulin-deficient diabetes. Type 2 diabetes is often associated with obesity and is characterized by impaired insulin secretion and insulin resistance. Additionally, a large group of other specific types of diabetes are recognized, including several forms of maturity-onset diabetes of youth (MODY), latent autoimmune diabetes of adults (LADA), type 1.5, genetic defects of insulin action, and various endocrinopathies. Another major category is gestational diabetes mellitus (GDM). It is expected that these classifications will be further refined as advances in genetic analysis and immunologic tests unfold (see Chapter 4, *Pathogenesis*).

TABLE 3.1 — Classification of Diabetes Mellitus

Type	Etiology	Genetics	Therapeutics
Type 1A	Autoimmune β-cell destruction	High-risk genetic markers confer increased susceptibility	Insulin
Type 1B	Nonautoimmune insulin deficiency and insulin resistance	Unknown, but autosomal dominant penetrance	Initially requires insulin, but occasionally can be controlled with oral agents
LADA	Autoimmune β-cell destruction (phenotypic type 1 diabetes)	High-risk genetic markers confer increased susceptibility	Insulin
Glucokinase MODY	Resetting of pancreatic glucose sensor	Mutation of glucokinase gene on chromosome 7	Often none or a sulfonylurea
Transcription factor MODY	Insulin secretory defect	Mutation of hepatocyte nuclear factor genes and insulin promoter factor gene	Sulfonylurea or insulin
Type 2	Insulin resistance and relative insulin deficiency	Likely polygenic	Sulfonylureas, α-glucosidase inhibitors, thiazolidinediones, insulin, metformin

Type 1.5	Insulin resistance (phenotypic type 2 diabetes) and insulin deficiency due to autoimmune β-cell destruction	Unknown	Unknown which therapies are best, but all available drugs likely work
Pancreatic diabetes	Insulin and glucagon deficiency	Variable—depends on etiology	Insulin, pancreatic enzymes
Lipodystrophic diabetes	Severe insulin resistance	Variable, based on whether congenital or acquired	Insulin sensitizers, insulin
Type 3 diabetes ("double diabetes")	Classic autoimmune β-cell destruction in childhood with later development of insulin resistance syndrome	Same high-risk genetic markers as seen in type 1 diabetes in addition to family history of obesity and/or type 2 diabetes	Insulin ± insulin sensitizer

Abbreviations: LADA, latent autoimmune diabetes of adults; MODY, mature-onset diabetes of youth.

Adapted from: Hirsch IB, Trence DL. *Optimizing Diabetes Care for the Practitioner*. Philadelphia, Pa: Lippincott Williams and Wilkins; 2003:6-7.

Impaired Glucose Tolerance and Impaired Fasting Glucose (Prediabetes)

In any given patient with diabetes mellitus, the degree of hyperglycemia may change over time. Depending on the extent of the underlying disease process, diabetes may be present but may not have progressed to the point of causing hyperglycemia. Interim stages of hyperglycemia include impaired glucose tolerance (IGT) and impaired fasting glucose (IFG), now called "prediabetes." In the absence of pregnancy, IGT and IFG are not clinical entities in their own right, but rather risk factors for current *and* future disease. They may be identified by an oral glucose tolerance test (OGTT) or an assessment of fasting plasma glucose (FPG). The latter method is preferred because of ease of use, acceptability to patients, and lower cost. IFG is present if FPG = 100 mg/dL to 125 mg/dL; IGT if 2-hour plasma glucose = 140 mg/dL to 199 mg/dL.

Type 1 Diabetes

Type 1 diabetes mellitus is characterized by cellular-mediated autoimmune destruction of the β cells of the pancreas. It is always associated with eventual absolute insulin deficiency and thus insulin is required to avoid diabetic ketoacidosis, which is associated with significant morbidity and mortality (see Chapter 13, *Acute Complications*). Markers of the immune destruction of the β cells include islet-cell autoantibodies (ICAs), autoantibodies to insulin (IAAs), autoantibodies to glutamic acid decarboxylase (GAD_{65}), and autoantibodies to the tyrosine phosphatases 1A-2 and 1A-2β (see Chapter 4, *Pathogenesis*). None of these antibodies appear to contribute to the etiology of β-cell destruction. However, their measurement helps to clarify the pathogenesis of diabetes in circumstances where the etiology is unclear. It should be mentioned that serum insulin (or C peptide) levels are not a good diagnostic tool for type 1 diabetes. Early in the course of the disease, especially in the case of LADA (see below), endogenous insulin secretion will be present and insulin secretion may be measurable for months or even years after diagnosis.

Autoimmune destruction of β cells likely results from the convergence of genetic and environmental factors that are as yet poorly defined. Although patients are not usually obese when they present with type 1 diabetes, the presence of obesity does not preclude the diagnosis. These patients are also prone to other autoimmune disorders such as Graves' disease, Hashimoto's thyroiditis, Addison's disease, vitiligo, celiac sprue, and pernicious anemia.

■ Idiopathic Diabetes (Type 1B)

Some forms of type 1 diabetes have no clear etiology. Patients with this type of diabetes, known as type 1B, may be permanently insulinopenic and prone to ketoacidosis but have no evidence of autoimmunity. Most are of Asian or African origin and present with intermittent episodes of ketoacidosis. Apart from these acute episodes, however, the degree of insulin deficiency varies. Type 1B diabetes is strongly inherited, lacks immunologic evidence of β-cell autoimmunity, and is not HLA associated. The need for insulin replacement therapy in affected patients may come and go.

Pancreatic Diabetes

Severe insulin deficiency also characterizes pancreatic diabetes, which is caused by diseases of the exocrine pancreas, such as pancreatitis, trauma, or pancreatectomy, or neoplasia. With the exception of cancer, damage to the pancreas must be significant for diabetes to occur. Automobile accidents, especially when the driver is not wearing a seatbelt, are a common cause of pancreatic diabetes, as the impact from the bottom of the steering wheel can crush the pancreas severely. If extensive enough, cystic fibrosis and hemochromatosis will also destroy β-cell mass.

Type 2 Diabetes

Patients with type 2 diabetes, which is outside the scope of this book, have insulin resistance and relative insulin deficiency. As type 2 diabetes progresses and oral antidiabetic agents lose their effectiveness, insulin replacement therapy may be necessary for treatment of hyperglycemia.

The etiology of this form of diabetes is multifactorial and only partially understood. Most people with type 2 diabetes are obese and have obesity-related insulin resistance. Unlike type 1 diabetes, autoimmune β-cell destruction does not play a role. Growing understanding of the causes will likely yield more definitive subclassifications of this disease in the future.

Type 2 diabetes is often associated with a strong genetic predisposition. Major acquired environmental risk factors include advancing age, obesity, and a sedentary lifestyle. Type 2 diabetes is also associated with hypertension, dyslipidemia, and central adiposity, and is more prevalent among Hispanics, African Americans, American Indians, Pacific Islanders, and Asian Americans. Women with a history of GDM, or who have given birth to an infant weighing >9 lb, are also at greater risk than the general population.

Ketoacidosis seldom occurs spontaneously in patients with type 2 diabetes, and its presence is usually associated with the stress of another illness, such as infection. When it does occur, it is usually as not as severe as in patients with type 1 diabetes, is more easily treated, and may be accompanied by hyperosmolar coma.

Typically, type 2 diabetes goes undiagnosed for many years because the classic symptoms of diabetes are seldom apparent in the early stages of disease development. Nevertheless, patients with type 2 diabetes are at premature risk for macrovascular complications associated with insulin resistance and the metabolic syndrome. Further, the risk for microvascular complications is similar to that of type 1 diabetes, depending on the duration and severity of hyperglycemia.

Maturity-Onset Diabetes of Youth

MODY is a heterogeneous group of autosomal dominantly inherited disorders marked by nonketotic onset of disease in childhood or adolescence and a primary defect in the function of pancreatic β cells. Glucokinase MODY (MODY-2) is a mild, nonprogressive hyperglycemia caused by resetting of the pancreatic glucose sensor. The mild fasting hyperglycemia (110 to 145 mg/dL) may be recognized as early as birth or discovered years later, usually by chance. All other MODY types fall into the category of transcription factor MODY. As the main defect affects insulin secretion, insulin secretagogues and insulin are primarily used for treatment, although other antidiabetic agents have not been formally studied. Information about the exact identification of MODY may be obtained at www.diabetesgenes.org.

Latent Autoimmune Diabetes of Adults and Type 1.5 Diabetes

LADA is not a designated category in the ADA report on the classification of diabetes, but the term is often used interchangeably in the literature with "type

1.5 diabetes." This has created confusion, but what is agreed upon is that all of these patients who develop diabetes later in life are positive to one of the islet cell antibodies.

■ LADA

One of the first reports of an autoimmune process causing a gradual-onset form of type 1 diabetes in adults appeared in 1994. The authors examined 19 of 65 patients who presented with "adult-onset" diabetes and who were deemed "insulin requiring." These adult patients were generally younger than the other study subjects (mean age, 57.2 ± 2.2 vs 63.5 ± 1.4 years, respectively [$P = 0.02$]), with their onset of diabetes occurring earlier (mean age at onset, 46.3 ± 2.3 vs 55.3 ± 1.4 years, respectively [$P = 0.002$]). They also had lower postprandial C peptide levels than the group not receiving insulin (1.3 ± 0.36 vs 4.6 ± 0.39 μg ml^{-1}, respectively [$P = <0.001$]). Notably, the frequency of GADs was 73.7% in the group receiving insulin compared with 4.3% in those not ($P = <0.001$). The conclusion from this study was that adults with newly diagnosed diabetes can have an autoimmune etiology leading to β-cell destruction and insulin deficiency. The pathogenesis of this form of diabetes is comparable to that seen in classic type 1 diabetes of children, except that the rate and extent of β-cell destruction in the adults appears to be more variable with slower β-cell destruction. Because of this slower progression and more variable presentation, diagnosis may be delayed or missed and inappropriate or ineffective treatment instituted.

■ Differentiating LADA from Type 1.5 Diabetes

Overweight LADA patients (with a body mass index of 27.3 kg/m^2) share both the phenotypic characteristics and the insulin resistance seen in patients with type 2 diabetes. Thus some prefer the use of the term

30

"type 1.5 diabetes" to classify these patients, although this classification is not official. Until a new classification system is developed, the differentiation between LADA and type 1.5 diabetes is as follows:

- Adults who develop diabetes, who are of normal body weight (body mass index <25 kg/m^2), and who are positive for one of the islet antibodies are generally considered to have LADA.
- Overweight patients with a body mass index >25 kg/m^2 who are likely to be insulin resistant and are positive for one of the islet antibodies are classified as having type 1.5 diabetes. Phenotypically, these patients are indistinguishable from those with classic type 2 diabetes.

Although this classification has many limitations, it assists in formulating treatment strategies until definitive studies are completed. In most cases of LADA, insulin therapy will need to be initiated. Although data regarding treatment of type 1.5 diabetes are scant, using an insulin sensitizer, insulin secretagogue, and/or insulin therapy soon after diagnosis may be warranted to address both the autoimmune attack on β cells and the insulin resistance.

Type 3 (Hybrid) and Lipodystrophic Diabetes

Type 3 diabetes, also called hybrid diabetes or double diabetes, is considered when the patient, usually a child, with classic type 1 diabetes develops insulin resistance later in life. Given that 25% of Americans are obese or suffer from the syndrome of insulin resistance, type 3 diabetes is not an unusual diagnosis. Women with type 1 diabetes may also develop polycystic ovarian syndrome normally associated with the insulin resistance of type 2 diabetes. These patients often respond well to insulin sensitizers, though there are few published data on this group. African Americans with type 3 diabetes have the typical autoimmunity found in type 1 diabetes and thus the diagnosis needs to be differentiated from idiopathic diabetes. Lipodystrophic diabetes, associated with lipodystrophies, is a syndrome of severe insulin resistance often with diabetes, hypertriglyceridemia, and fatty liver. Selective but variable loss of fat tissue characterizes this form of diabetes, with the degree of severity depending on the amount of fat loss. Both familial and acquired lipodystrophic diabetes have been identified, and these patients may require hundreds of units of insulin per day to achieve glycemic control.

Gestational Diabetes Mellitus

GDM occurring in pregnant women is defined as any degree of glucose intolerance with onset or first recognition during pregnancy, regardless of whether insulin or only diet modification is the prescribed treatment or whether the condition persists after pregnancy. Additionally, it does not exclude the possibility that glucose intolerance may have existed unrecognized before pregnancy or begun concomitantly with pregnancy. Six weeks or more after pregnancy ends, the patient should be reclassified into one of the following categories: diabetes, IFG, IGT, or normoglycemia. In the majority of cases, glucose regulation will return to normal after delivery. Most cases of diabetes discovered during pregnancy are type 2; however, initial presentation of type 1 diabetes may occur as well.

SUGGESTED READING

American Diabetes Association. Diagnosis and classification of diabetes mellitus. *Diabetes Care*. 2005;28(suppl 1):S37-S42.

American Diabetes Association. Standards of medical care in diabetes. *Diabetes Care*. 2005;28(suppl 1):S4-S36.

Eisenbarth GS. Classification, diagnostic tests, and pathogenesis of type 1 diabetes mellitus. In: Becker KL, ed. *Principles and Practice of Endocrinology and Metabolism*. 3rd ed. Philadelphia, Pa: Lippincott Williams and Wilkins; 2001.

Fajans SS, Bell GI, Polonsky KS. Molecular mechanisms and clinical pathophysiology of maturity-onset diabetes of the young. *N Engl J Med*. 2001;345:971-980.

Garg A. Lipodystrophies. *Am J Med*. 2000;108:143-152.

Juneja R, Palmer JP. Type 1½ diabetes: myth or reality? *Autoimmunity*. 1999;29:65-83.

Palmer JP, Hirsch IB. What's in a name: latent autoimmune diabetes of adults, type 1.5, adult-onset, and type 1 diabetes. *Diabetes Care*. 2003;26:536-538.

4 Pathogenesis

Type 1 diabetes is characterized by autoimmune β-cell destruction resulting from genetic, environmental, and immunologic factors. In genetically susceptible individuals, β-cell mass is normal at birth but progressively deteriorates over a period of months to years (**Figure 4.1**). Immunologists often refer to the immune-mediated form of this disease, characterized by the presence of anti-islet autoantibodies, as type 1A diabetes in order to distinguish it from type 1B, or idiopathic, insulin-deficient diabetes. It is largely believed that the autoimmune destruction is triggered by infectious or environmental factors and sustained by a β-cell–specific molecule, and that certain immunologic markers emerge after the triggering event but before diabetes becomes clinically apparent. During this prodrome, insulin secretion becomes increasingly more compromised as β-cell mass diminishes, although it may take some time for glucose tolerance to be affected.

The clinical characteristics of diabetes do not become evident until the vast majority of β cells (approximately 80%) have been destroyed, at which point glucose intolerance occurs. The transition from glucose intolerance to overt diabetes often coincides with circumstances that increase the demand for insulin, such as illness, puberty, and pregnancy. This initial clinical presentation may then be followed by a brief "honeymoon period," during which time endogenous insulin production from residual β-cell function is enough to require only modest doses of exogenous insulin for glycemic control. Eventually, however, further destruction of the β cells by the autoimmune

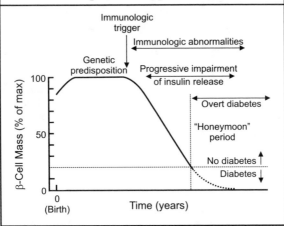

FIGURE 4.1 — Stages in the Development of Type 1 Diabetes

Individuals with a genetic predisposition are exposed to an immunologic trigger that sets off an autoimmune cascade, resulting in a gradual decline in β-cell mass. The downward slope of the β-cell mass varies among individuals. This progressive impairment in insulin resistance results in diabetes when ~80% of the β-cell mass is destroyed. A "honeymoon" period may be seen in the first 1 or 2 years after the onset of diabetes and is associated with reduced insulin requirements.

Adapted from: Skyler JS, ed, for the American Diabetes Association. *Medical Management of Type 1 Diabetes*. 3rd ed. New York, NY: The McGraw-Hill Companies; 1998.

process leads to complete insulin deficiency and the need for total insulin replacement.

Risk of Developing the Disease

Markers of immune destruction of β cells include islet-cell autoantibodies (ICAs), which are a composite of several different antibodies (eg, glutamic acid decarboxylase [GAD], insulin, IA-2/ICA512, and islet ganglioside) directed at pancreatic islet molecules. One, if not more, of these autoantibodies is present in 85% to 90% of individuals at the time fasting hyperglycemia is first detected. Also, type 1 diabetes has strong HLA associations, with linkage to the DQA and B genes, and is also influenced by the DRB genes. These HLA-DR/DQ alleles can be either predisposing or protective (**Table 4.1**).

Although type 1 diabetes is clearly linked to certain genotypes, most individuals with these haplotypes do not develop the disease, and many patients with type 1 diabetes do not have a first-degree relative with the disease. Nevertheless, the overall risk for developing type 1 diabetes in North American white siblings, parents, and children of patients with type 1 diabetes ranges from 1% to 15% compared with 0.12% in the general population (**Table 4.2**). Persons who are HLA-identical to a sibling with diabetes have approximately a 1:10 to 1:20 chance of developing diabetes, whereas siblings without these haplotypes in common have a <1:100 chance. Not all diabetic siblings express identical HLA haplotypes, however, possibly owing to the relatively large number of parents (20%) who are potentially homozygous for diabetogenic major histocompatibility complex (MHC) genes. Such a high proportion of homozygous parents is suggested by the finding that 5% of parents of offspring with type 1 diabetes develop overt disease, and that penetrance even in HLA-identical siblings is <1:4.

Environmental Factors

Given that identical twins do not necessarily develop type 1 diabetes in tandem, it is thought that environmental factors play a role in triggering the disease. Congenital rubella has been implicated as a possible contributing factor, since as many as 20% of children infected with the virus *in utero* later develop

TABLE 4.1 — Effect of Human Leukocyte Antigen Alleles on Susceptibility to Type 1 Diabetes Mellitus

DQ Alleles	Effect	Associated DR Class
A1*0301, B1*0302	Susceptible	DR4
A1*0501, B1*0201	Susceptible	DR3
A1*0101, B1*0501	Susceptible	DR1
A1*0301, B1*0201	Susceptible (African Americans)	DR7
A1*0102, B1*0502	Susceptible (Sardinians)	DR2 (DR16)
A1*0301, B1*0303	Susceptible (Japanese)	DR4
A1*0301, B1*0303	Susceptible (Japanese)	DR9
A1*0102, B1*0602	Protective	DR2 (DR15)
A1*0501, B1*0301	Protective	DR5
? B1*0600	Neutral	DR6

A1*0201, B1*0201	Neutral	DR7
A1*0301, B1*0303	Neutral	DR4
A1*0301, B1*0301	Neutral	DR4

Pietropaolo M, Trucco M. In: Le Roith D, et al, eds. *Diabetes Mellitus. A Fundamental and Clinical Text.* Philadelphia, Pa: Lippincott Williams and Wilkins; 2000:399-410.

TABLE 4.2 — Empiric Risk of Type 1 Diabetes Mellitus (T1DM)	
Group at Risk	**Empiric Risk (%)**
First-degree relatives of T1DM probands*	5-7[‡]
Individuals without relatives with T1DM*	<1
Children of affected father[†]	~6
Children of affected mother[†]	~2
* Estimates for North American white populations. † Estimates for Scandinavian populations. ‡ 1% to 15% range depending on the populations.	
Pietropaolo M, et al. *Clin Cornerstone.* 2001;4:1-16.	

the disease. These children express HLA alleles DR3 and DR4 and often have thyroiditis and other immunologic disorders in association with an abnormal T-lymphocyte phenotype. No other epidemiologically defined environmental factors have been clearly associated with type 1A diabetes.

Viral infections, particularly those occurring around the initial manifestation of diabetes, are known to precipitate hyperglycemia (secondary to insulin resistance associated with infection), but they do not play a primary role in pathogenesis. Coxsackievirus B4, which aroused interest after it was isolated from the pancreas of a child with recent-onset diabetes, is no longer considered a contributing factor because the same pancreas had multiple A and D cell islets, indicating chronic β-cell destruction prior to the viral infection. Because of the progressive nature of type 1 diabetes, any effort to identify environmental triggers of autoimmunity should focus on factors introduced months or years before, rather than immediately prior to, disease onset.

Immunologic Markers

Autoimmune diseases such as type 1 diabetes often feature a T-cell and humoral response against multiple target antigens. As autoimmunity in type 1 diabetes progresses from initial activation to a chronic condition, there is often an increase in the number of islet cell autoantigens targeted by T cells and antibodies. Immunologic diagnosis of type 1 diabetes is possible through the use of immunologic assays that detect autoantibodies to islet antigens in serum. Some assays for ICAs, ie, GAD, insulin, a molecule termed IA-2/ICA512, and ganglioside GM2-1, have sufficient specificity to identify persons at high risk for type 1 diabetes. Recently developed biochemical assays using recombinant human proteins to measure antibodies to insulin, GAD, and ICA512 show that >98% of patients with new-onset type 1 diabetes and prediabetes express at least one antibody, and >80% express two or more. These assays are more reliable than cytoplasmic islet cell antibody testing in both the diagnosis and prediction of type 1 diabetes.

Approximately 3% to 4% of first-degree relatives of individuals with type 1 diabetes have positive results on screening assays for ICAs. In these individuals, intravenous (IV) glucose-tolerance testing can be used to evaluate first-phase insulin release as an indicator of subclinical β-cell dysfunction. The loss of first-phase insulin secretion, as well as its rate of decline, helps to predict the time of onset of overt diabetes. For patients with initially normal insulin release, IV glucose-tolerance testing should be performed again in 3 to 6 months and, depending on its stability, every 3 to 12 months thereafter. Individuals with abnormal results should be alerted to their risk of developing type 1 diabetes and encouraged to monitor blood glucose regularly. Formulas have been developed to assist in this prediction process.

Preventive Therapy

A number of interventions have successfully delayed or prevented diabetes in animal models. Some have targeted the immune system directly (immunosuppression, selective T-cell subset deletion, induction of immunologic to islet proteins), whereas others have prevented islet-cell degradation by blocking cytotoxic cytokines or increasing islet resistance to destruction. Though results in animal models are promising, these interventions have been largely ineffective in preventing type 1A diabetes in humans. Because of the toxic side effects of immunosuppression, most trials examining the prevention of type 1 diabetes or amelioration of β-cell loss once the disease process is under way concentrate on nonimmunosuppressive strategies.

Recently, the Diabetes Prevention Trial—Type 1 Diabetes (DPT-1) was undertaken to determine whether insulin therapy could delay or prevent diabetes in nondiabetic relatives of patients with diabetes. In this randomized, controlled trial, 339 ICA positive first- and second-degree relatives of patients with type 1 diabetes were randomly assigned to undergo either close observation or an intervention that consisted of low-dose subcutaneous Ultralente insulin administered twice daily. Oral glucose tolerance tests were performed every 6 months for 3.7 years for the purpose of diagnosing diabetes. In contrast to smaller pilot studies showing prophylactic insulin therapy to be of value, the annualized rate of progression to diabetes in this larger study was 15.1% in the intervention group and 14.6% in the observation group. Among the explanations for this disappointing result were that intervention may have been too late or the dose of insulin too low to prevent or retard disease progression. Another large trial, the European Nicotinamide Diabetes Intervention Trial (ENDIT), was conducted to determine whether an amide of nicotinic acid, nicotinamide, which has been shown to have a protective effect on rodent β cells, can prevent or delay clinical onset of type 1 diabetes in ICA positive individuals with a first-degree family history of type 1 diabetes. Like the DPT-1, results of the ENDIT were negative.

Associated Autoimmune Disease

Approximately 20% of patients with type 1 diabetes develop other organ-specific autoimmune disease, such as celiac disease, hypothyroidism, Graves' disease, and pernicious anemia. Multiple disorders may be present in some patients as the result of two inherited polyendocrine autoimmune syndromes (type I and type II).

The type I syndrome usually manifests in infancy, with hypoparathyroidism, mucocutaneous candidiasis, and later, Addison's disease, as well as other organ-specific disorders. Fifteen percent of these children develop type 1 diabetes. This disorder is inherited in an autosomal recessive manner with no HLA association due to mutations of a gene (AIRE) located on chromosome 21. This mutated gene codes for an NDA-binding protein that is expressed in the thymus.

The type II polyendocrine autoimmune syndrome (Addison's disease, type 1 diabetes [50% of patients], Graves' disease, hypothyroidism, myasthenia gravis, and other organ-specific diseases) is strongly linked to HLA and can appear anytime from late childhood to early middle age. Undiagnosed organ-specific autoimmune disease is often familial and, at minimum, thyroid function tests should be performed in the first-degree relatives of these patients. Biochemical analysis for adrenal insufficiency and pernicious anemia should be undertaken in the event of suggestive symptoms or signs (eg, decreasing insulin requirements can herald the development of Addison's disease in a patient with type 1 diabetes before electrolyte abnormalities or hyperpigmentation develops). Autoantibody assays can aid in the detection of Addison's disease (21-hydroxylase autoantibodies) or celiac disease (transglutaminase autoantibodies) in patients with type 1 diabetes.

SUGGESTED READING

American Diabetes Association. Diagnosis and classification of diabetes mellitus. *Diabetes Care.* 2005;28(suppl 1):S37-S42.

American Diabetes Association. Standards of medical care in diabetes. *Diabetes Care.* 2005;28(suppl 1):S4-S36.

Atkinson MA, Naclaren NK. The pathogenesis of insulin-dependent diabetes mellitus. *N Engl J Med.* 1994;331:1428-1436.

Diabetes Prevention Trial—Type 1 Diabetes Study Group. Effects of insulin in relatives of patients with type 1 diabetes mellitus. *N Engl J Med.* 2002;346:1685-1691.

Eisenbarth GS. Classification, diagnostic tests, and pathogenesis of type 1 diabetes mellitus. In: Becker KL, ed. *Principles and Practice of Endocrinology and Metabolism.* 3rd ed. Philadelphia, Pa: Lippincott Williams and Wilkins; 2001.

Gale EA, European Nicotinamide Diabetes Intervention Trial Group. Intervening before the onset of type 1 diabetes: baseline data from the European Nicotinamide Diabetes Intervention Trial (ENDIT). *Diabetologia.* 2003;46:339-346.

Kruglyak L, Lander ES. Complete multipoint sib-pair analysis of qualitative and quantitative traits. *Am J Hum Genet.* 1995;57:439-454.

Liu E, Eisenbarth GS. Type 1A diabetes mellitus–associated autoimmunity. *Endocrinol Metab Clin North Am.* 2002;31:391-410.

Pietropaolo M, Trucco M. Major histocompatibility locus and other genes that determine the risk of development of type 1 diabetes mellitus. In: Le Roith D, Taylor SI, Olefsky JM, eds. *Diabetes Mellitus. A Fundamental and Clinical Text.* Philadelphia, Pa: Lippincott Williams and Wilkins; 2000:399-410.

5 Diagnosis

The diagnosis of diabetes mellitus may be made on the basis of classic symptoms and clear elevation on more than one fasting or postprandial glucose level. Although this chapter refers to the two broad etiopathogenic categories of diabetes mellitus, type 1 and type 2, as well as gestational diabetes mellitus (GDM), many diabetic individuals do not easily fit into a single class. Thus once a diagnosis of diabetes is established, it is necessary to understand the underlying etiology and pathogenesis of the disease (see Chapter 3, *Classification* and Chapter 4, *Pathogenesis*) to determine the most effective treatment.

Diagnostic Criteria

Patients with type 1 diabetes typically present with polyuria, polydipsia, polyphasia, and unexplained weight loss. Less often, the initial symptom is severe ketoacidosis, manifesting as nausea, vomiting, and sometimes coma.

In addition to these symptoms, the diagnosis is based on one of three tests:

- Random plasma glucose testing
- Fasting plasma glucose (FPG) concentration
- A properly performed oral glucose tolerance test (OGTT), although the OGTT is not typically needed for routine clinical use.

The criteria for diagnosis of diabetes are shown in **Table 5**.**1**. Each of the three methods listed must be confirmed on a subsequent day to make a definitive diagnosis. For example, symptoms together with a ca-

**TABLE 5.1 — Criteria for the
Diagnosis of Diabetes Mellitus**

Symptoms of diabetes plus casual plasma glucose concentration ≥200 mg/dL (11.1 mmol/L). Casual is defined as any time of day without regard to time since last meal. The classic symptoms of diabetes include polyuria, polydipsia, and unexplained weight loss.

or

FPG ≥126 mg/dL (7.0 mmol/L). Fasting is defined as no caloric intake for at least 8 hours.

or

2-hour PG ≥200 mg/dL (11.1 mmol/dL) during an OGTT. The test should be performed using a glucose load containing the equivalent of 75 g anhydrous glucose dissolved in water.

In the absence of unequivocal hyperglycemia with acute metabolic decompensation, these criteria should be confirmed by repeat testing on a different day. The third measure (OGTT) is not recommended for routine clinical use.

Abbreviations: FPG, fasting plasma glucose; PG, plasma glucose; OGTT, oral glucose tolerance test.

Adapted from: American Diabetes Association. *Diabetes Care.* 2005;28(suppl 1):S37-S42.

sual plasma glucose ≥200 mg/dL (11.1 mmol/L), must be confirmed on a subsequent day by:

- An FPG ≥126 mg/dL (7.0 mmol/L)
- An OGTT with the 2-hour postload value ≥200 mg/dL (11.1 mmol/L)
- Symptoms with a casual plasma glucose ≥200 mg/dL (11.1 mmol/L).

These diagnostic tests are also of value in identifying patients whose glucose levels do meet the diagnostic criteria for diabetes but are still too high to be considered normal. Such individuals are considered to have impaired fasting glucose (IFG) if FPG is used for testing, or impaired glucose tolerance (IGT) if OGTT is used. These conditions are often referred to as "pre-diabetes," defined as FPG levels $\geq$100 mg/dL (5.6 mmol/L) but <126 mg/dL (7.0 mmol/L) or 2-hour values in the OGTT of $\geq$140 mg/dL (7.8 mmol/L) but <200 mg/dL (11.1 mmol/L). Patients with prediabetes are at greater risk for overt diabetes and cardiovascular disease. Because a finding of impaired glucose homeostasis will be more likely if the 2-hour OGTT cutoff of 140 mg/dL (7.8 mmol/L) is used rather than the fasting cutoff of 100 mg/dL (5.6 mmol/L), it is important that the clinician always report which test was used. The categories of FPG and OGTT are listed in **Table 5.2**. The FPG is considered the most reliable and convenient test for diagnosing diabetes in asymptomatic individuals.

Glycosylated hemoglobin (A1C) assays are not used to diagnose diabetes because they are not sensitive enough, ie, a value in the normal range is not sufficient to rule out the presence of diabetes. Moreover, they are not standardized countrywide. It is hoped that these problems will be addressed so that the A1C value can be used efficiently and accurately for diagnostic purposes. It should be noted, however, that an A1C value above the normal range is strongly predictive of diabetes.

■ Differentiating Between Type 1 and Type 2 Diabetes

In general, type 1 diabetes can be differentiated from type 2 based on a number of factors:

- Type 1 diabetes tends to be diagnosed before age 30 years, and type 2 after age 30 years—however, type 1 diabetes can occur at virtually any age, and the number of children with type 2 diabetes is growing at an alarming rate.

**TABLE 5.2 — Diagnostic Categories
of Fasting Plasma Glucose and
Oral Glucose Tolerance Test**

Fasting Plasma Glucose
- FPG <100 mg/dL (5.6 mmol/L) = normal fasting glucose
- FPG 100-125 mg/dL (5.6-6.9 mmol/L) = impaired fasting glucose
- FPG ≥126 mg/dL (7.0 mmol/L) = provisional diagnosis of diabetes (the diagnosis must be confirmed, as described in text)

Oral Glucose Tolerance Test
- 2-hour postload glucose (2-h PG) <140 mg/dL (7.8 mmol/L) = normal glucose tolerance
- 2-h PG 140-199 mg/dL (7.8-11.1 mmol/L) = impaired glucose tolerance
- 2-h PG ≥200 (11.1 mmol/L) = provisional diagnosis of diabetes (the diagnosis must be confirmed, as described in text)

Abbreviations: FPG, fasting plasma glucose; PG, plasma glucose.

American Diabetes Association. *Diabetes Care.* 2005;28(suppl 1):S37-S42.

- Whereas most patients with type 1 diabetes tend to be lean, patients with type 2 are generally (but not always) centrally obese.
- Most patients with type 2 have a family history of diabetes while most with type 1 do not.
- Most patients with type 1 diabetes have experienced symptoms such as polyuria, polydipsia, and weight loss before presentation, whereas most patients with type 2 are asymptomatic or only mildly symptomatic at presentation.
- Many patients with type 2 diabetes present with acanthosis nigricans, a brown-to-black hyperpigmentation of the skin.

- Patients with type 2 diabetes commonly have the metabolic syndrome (obesity, hypertension, dyslipidemia, and insulin resistance) at the time of diagnosis, whereas patients with type 1 diabetes do not.
- Glutamic acid decarboxylase (GAD) antibodies are present in type 1 diabetes but not in type 2 diabetes.
- If glucose toxicity is not present, C peptide and insulin levels are usually high in people with newly diagnosed type 2 diabetes; C peptide values are usually low in patients with type 1 diabetes, unless they are measured during the honeymoon period.

Gestational Diabetes Mellitus Testing

In the past, testing for GDM was performed routinely in all pregnancies. However, screening is no longer recommended for pregnant women who meet *all* of the following criteria:
- <25 years of age
- Normal body weight
- No family history of diabetes (ie, first-degree relative)
- No history of abnormal glucose metabolism or poor obstetric outcome
- Not member of an ethnic/racial group with a high prevalence of diabetes (eg, Hispanic American, Native American, Asian American, African American, Pacific Islander).

Women who meet these criteria are considered to be at low risk for the development of glucose intolerance during pregnancy.

Women with clinical characteristics indicating a high risk for GDM (marked obesity, personal history of GDM, glycosuria, or a strong family history of GDM) should be identified at the first prenatal visit and undergo diagnostic testing as soon as possible. If GDM is not present, another test should be performed between 24 weeks and 28 weeks of gestation. Women at average risk also should be tested at 24 to 28 weeks of gestation.

The diagnosis of GDM is based on an OGTT (**Table 5.3**). However, women who meet the plasma glucose criteria in **Table 5.1** do not require a glucose challenge test (GCT). Those at average or high risk for GDM may be evaluated in one of two ways:

- *One-step approach*: Perform a diagnostic OGTT without prior plasma or serum glucose screening. This one-step approach may be cost-effective in high-risk patients or populations (eg, Native Americans).
- *Two-step approach*: Screen initially by measuring the plasma or serum glucose concentration 1 hour after a 50-g oral glucose load; women who exceed the glucose threshold value on the GCT should then undergo a diagnostic OGTT. When this two-step approach is used, a glucose threshold value >140 mg/dL (7.8 mmol/L) identifies approximately 80% of women with GDM, and this proportion is increased to 90% when the cutoff is established at >130 mg/dL (7.2 mmol/L).

Alternatively, the diagnosis can be made using a 75-g glucose load and the glucose threshold values listed for fasting, 1 hour, and 2 hours (**Table 5.3**); however, this procedure is not as well validated as the 100-g OGTT.

TABLE 5.3 — Diagnosis of Gestational Diabetes Mellitus With a 100-g or 75-g Glucose Load

Glucose Load	mg/dL	mmol/L
100-g		
Fasting	95	5.3
1-hour	180	10.0
2-hour	155	8.6
3-hour	140	7.8
75-g		
Fasting	95	5.3
1-hour	180	10.0
2-hour	155	8.6

Two or more of the venous plasma concentrations must be met or exceeded for a positive diagnosis. The test should be done in the morning after an overnight fast of between 8 and 14 hours and after at least 3 days of unrestricted diet (carbohydrate $\geq$150 g/day) and unlimited physical activity. The subject should remain seated and should not smoke throughout the test.

American Diabetes Association. *Diabetes Care*. 2005;28(suppl 1):S37-S42.

Screening Asymptomatic Individuals

■ Type 1 Diabetes

Type 1 diabetes is typified by numerous autoantibodies to protein epitopes on the surface of or within the β cells of the pancreas. The detection of such markers (eg, islet-cell autoantibodies [ICA], autoantibodies to insulin [IAA], GAD, 1A-2) before the development of overt disease can identify patients at risk. However, clinical testing of individuals for these autoantibodies is not recommended owing to the lack of established cutoff values for some assays in the clinical setting, as well as the absence of consensus on what action should be taken in the event of a positive result. On the other hand, autoantibody testing may be warranted

when there is uncertainty as to whether newly diagnosed patients have immune-mediated type 1 diabetes.

■ Type 2 Diabetes

Because type 2 diabetes has a more insidious onset than type 1 diabetes, it is likely to be discovered
during a screening test or when one of its complications is detected. Indeed, it is estimated that in the
United States approximately 5.4 million cases, or one
third of all diabetes, is undiagnosed. There is evidence
that patients with retinopathy at the time of diagnosis
are likely to have been glucose intolerant for at least
6.5 years; and people with type 2 diabetes are more
apt to develop premature macrovascular disease because of its association with insulin resistance, which
may be present for as many as 10 to 15 years before
diabetes is officially diagnosed. In fact, it is not uncommon for patients to present with type 2 diabetes
at the time of their first stroke or heart attack. Early
detection is therefore considered essential to relieving
the burden of type 2 diabetes and its complications.
Suggested criteria for testing presumably healthy individuals for diabetes are listed in **Table 5.4**.

SUGGESTED READING

American Diabetes Association. Diagnosis and classification of
diabetes mellitus. *Diabetes Care*. 2005;28(suppl 1):S37-S42.

American Diabetes Association. Standards of medical care in diabetes. *Diabetes Care*. 2005;28(suppl 1):S4-S36.

Genuth S, Alberti KG, Bennett P, et al. Follow-up report on the
diagnosis of diabetes mellitus. *Diabetes Care*. 2003;26:3160-3167.

TABLE 5.4 — Criteria for Testing for Diabetes in Asymptomatic, Undiagnosed Individuals

- Testing for diabetes should be considered in individuals at age ≥45 years, particularly in those with a BMI ≥25 kg/m^2*; if normal, it should be repeated at 3-year intervals.
- Testing should be considered at a younger age or be carried out more frequently in individuals who are overweight (BMI >25 kg/m^2*) and have additional risk factors:
  - A first-degree relative with diabetes
  - Habitually physically inactive
  - Member of a high-risk ethnic population (eg, African American, Hispanic American, Native American, Asian American, Pacific Islander)
  - Given birth to an infant weighing >9 lb or have been diagnosed with gestational diabetes mellitus
  - Hypertension (≥140/90 mm Hg)
  - HDL cholesterol level <35 mg/dL (0.90 mmol/L) and/or a triglyceride level >250 mg/dL (2.82 mmol/L)
  - Polycystic ovary syndrome
  - On previous testing, had impaired glucose tolerance or impaired fasting glucose
  - A history of vascular disease.

Abbreviations: BMI, body mass index; HDL, high-density lipoprotein.

The oral glucose tolerance test or fasting plasma glucose test may be used to diagnose diabetes; however, in clinical settings the fasting plasma glucose test is greatly preferred because of ease of administration, convenience, acceptability to patients, and lower cost.

* May not be correct for all ethnic groups.

Adapted from: American Diabetes Association. *Diabetes Care.* 2005;28(suppl 1):S4-S36.

6　Glycemic Goals

The important benefits of achieving near-normal glycemic control in diabetes management were first demonstrated in the Diabetes Control and Complications Trial, a landmark study completed in 1993. The trial showed definitively that stringent blood glucose control can postpone, prevent, or slow the progression of retinal, renal, and neurologic complications in individuals with type 1 diabetes. In patients treated with intensive therapy—that is, therapy aimed at keeping blood glucose levels as close to normal as possible—the risk of developing diabetic retinopathy was reduced by 76%, diabetic neuropathy by 60%, and diabetic nephropathy by 54%, compared with conventionally treated patients. Other benefits of intensive diabetes management include improved lipid profiles, reduced risk factors for macrovascular disease, and better maternal and fetal health (**Table 6.1**).

Patients with type 1 diabetes require multiple daily injections or an insulin pump to achieve and maintain near-normal glycemia. Because this therapeutic approach entails matching insulin regimens to carbohydrate intake, physical activity, and other variables, a physician-coordinated team should work with the patient to devise an individualized management program reflecting the patient's age, school or work situation, physical activity, eating patterns, social and cultural influences, and the presence of diabetic complications or other medical conditions. The management team usually consists of nurses, dieticians, pharmacists, and mental health professionals, although other specialists may be consulted as needed. In all cases, it is essential that individuals with diabetes be encouraged to

TABLE 6.1 — Benefits of Intensive Diabetes Management

- Lowered risk of microvascular complications developing and/or progressing
- More predictable blood glucose values
- Probably lowering of risk of macrovascular complications
- Improved plasma lipid levels and leukocyte function
- Lowered maternal and fetal morbidity and/or mortality during pregnancy
- Diminished risk of congenital malformations in the fetus
- Optimal linear growth in children
- Better control of the dawn phenomenon
- A feeling of physical and emotional well-being and of "being in control"
- Greater freedom of lifestyle and daily schedule
- Greater understanding of diabetes care

Adapted from: Klingensmith GJ, ed. *Intensive Diabetes Management*. 3rd ed. Alexandria, Va: American Diabetes Association; 2003:3.

assume an active role in their own care. The management plan should be established collaboratively and agreed upon by the patient, the patient's family, and the health care team.

While intensive diabetes management is the preferred therapeutic approach for most patients with type 1 diabetes, the goals of therapy may be adjusted for some patients whose individual circumstances render the risks of intensive management greater than the benefits. Contraindications to intensive diabetes management include limited life expectancy, very young or very old age, hypoglycemia unawareness, advanced complications, and comorbid conditions. Potentially dangerous hypoglycemia and weight gain are the leading adverse effects.

Setting and Assessing Goals

A fundamental component of planning and evaluating therapy is setting reasonable goals. Although patients should be made aware of optimal glycemic goals at the first office visit, establishing a short-term intermediate goal may be more acceptable. For example, the patient who presents with a glucose level of 300 mg/dL might strive for an initial goal of all values <200 mg/dL. Recommended glycemic goals for adults are listed in **Table 6.2**. Severe or frequent hypoglycemia is an indication for the modification of treatment regimens, including setting higher glycemic goals.

Glycosylated Hemoglobin

An important tool for monitoring long-term glycemic control is the glycosylated hemoglobin (A1C) test. Hemoglobin exposed to glucose in the bloodstream slowly becomes nonenzymatically bound to glucose in a concentration-dependent fashion. The percentage of hemoglobin molecules that are glycosylated (bound to glucose) indicates what the average blood glucose concentration has been over the life of the cell. As such, determining the A1C value provides an objective assessment of overall glycemic control over the preceding 2 to 3 months. Additionally, it serves to verify the accuracy of the patient's reported blood glucose results (see below) and the adequacy of the blood glucose testing schedule.

A1C tests should be performed every 3 months to assess whether the desired level of glycemic control has been achieved and maintained. Monthly measurements may be warranted during periods of changing diabetes regimens. The significance of the test results should be discussed with the patient, along with goals that are deemed safe and yet ultimately reduce the risk

TABLE 6.2 — Glycemic Goals for Adults Patients With Diabetes	
Index	**Goal**
A1C	<7.0%*
Preprandial plasma glucose	90-130 mg/dL (5.0-7.2 mmol/L)
Peak postprandial plasma glucose	<180 mg/dL (10.0 mmol/L)

Key concepts in setting goals:
- Goals should be individualized
- Certain populations (children, pregnant women, and elderly) require special considerations
- Less intensive glycemic goals may be indicated in patients with severe or frequent hypoglycemia
- More intensive glycemic goals may further reduce microvascular complications at the cost of increasing hypoglycemia
- Postprandial glucose may be targeted if A1C goals are not met despite reaching preprandial goals

Abbreviation: AIC, glycosylated hemoglobin.

* Referenced to a nondiabetic range of 4.0% to 6.0% using a Diabetes Control and Complications Trial–based assay.

Adapted from: American Diabetes Association. *Diabetes Care*. 2005;28(suppl 1):S4-S36.

of long-term complications. The American Association of Clinical Endocrinologists calls for establishing A1C as the primary method of evaluating glycemic control, with the target value <6.5% (below the American Diabetes Association-endorsed goal of <7%). A realistic target is the lowest A1C possible without unacceptable levels of hypoglycemia, with action recommended when A1C levels are persistently >7%.

Self-Monitoring of Blood Glucose

Self-monitoring of blood glucose (SMBG), discussed extensively in Chapter 10, *Monitoring Glycemic Status* and Chapter 11, *Using Blood Glucose Data Technology for Pattern Management*, is an essential aspect of intensive glycemic control. SMBG enables patients to:

- Evaluate their individual response to therapy
- Assess whether glycemic targets are being met
- Prevent hypoglycemia
- Adjust medications, diet, and physical activity.

6

A person with type 1 diabetes practicing intensive diabetes management may test blood glucose levels 4 to 6 times per day, usually before meals and at bedtime. When adding to or modifying therapy, patients should test more often than usual.

Glycemic Goals During Pregnancy

Gestational diabetes mellitus (GDM) is defined as any degree of glucose intolerance with onset or first recognition during pregnancy (see Chapter 5, *Diagnosis*). It is associated with increased frequency of maternal hypertensive disorders and cesarean delivery as the result of fetal growth disorders and/or modified obstetric management. Additionally, the presence of fasting hyperglycemia (>105 mg/dL) may increase the risk of intrauterine fetal death during the last 1 to 2 months of gestation. Although uncomplicated GDM with mild fasting hyperglycemia is not associated with increased perinatal mortality, it can increase the risk of fetal macrosomia.

Maternal metabolic monitoring should be directed at detecting hyperglycemia severe enough to increase risk to the fetus. Action should be taken if SMBG results are *not* maintained at the following levels:

- Fasting whole blood glucose: ≤95 mg/dL (5.3 mmol/L)
- Fasting plasma glucose: ≤105 mg/dL (5.8 mmol/L)

or

- 1-hour postprandial whole blood glucose: ≤140 mg/dL (7.8 mmol/L)
- 1-hour postprandial plasma glucose: ≤155 mg/dL (8.6 mmol/L)

or

- 2-hour postprandial whole blood glucose: ≤120 mg/dL (6.7 mmol/L)
- 2-hour postprandial plasma glucose: ≤130 mg/dL (7.2 mmol/L)

Glucose levels should be checked before and 1 hour after meals, at bedtime, and at 2:00 AM to 3:00 AM and insulin dosages adjusted daily. Ideal goals of therapy are plasma glucose levels of 63 to 75 mg/dL before meals (capillary 55 to 65 mg/dL) and <140 mg/dL 1 hour following meals (capillary <120 mg/dL). Target A1C is <7.0%.

SUGGESTED READING

American Diabetes Association. Diagnosis and classification of diabetes mellitus. *Diabetes Care*. 2005;28(suppl 1):S37-S42.

American Diabetes Association. Standards of medical care in diabetes. *Diabetes Care*. 2005;28(suppl 1):S4-S36.

The Diabetes Control and Complications Trial Research Group. The effect of intensive treatment of diabetes on the development and progression of long-term complications in insulin-dependent diabetes mellitus. *N Engl J Med*. 1993;329:977-986.

Hirsch IB, Trence DL. *Optimizing Diabetes Care for the Practitioner*. Philadelphia, Pa: Lippincott Williams and Wilkins; 2003.

Klingensmith GJ, ed. *Intensive Diabetes Management*. 3rd ed. Alexandria, Va: American Diabetes Association; 2003.

7 Nonpharmacologic Management

Medical Nutrition Therapy

Medical nutrition therapy (MNT), which entails modifying nutritional intake to achieve and maintain glycemic goals, is a vital component of type 1 diabetes management. The specific goals of MNT are:

- Maintaining blood glucose levels as near normal as possible by balancing food intake with insulin and physical activity
- Achieving optimal serum lipid and blood pressure levels
- Providing adequate calories for maintaining or attaining a reasonable weight for adults and normal growth in children or meeting the increased metabolic needs of pregnancy or illness
- Preventing or treating the acute and chronic complications of diabetes
- Promoting overall health
- Addressing individual nutritional needs.

Establishing specific nutrition-related goals requires a team approach that actively involves the person with diabetes. Because of the interplay between nutrition intake, medication, and exercise in determining blood glucose levels, a registered dietitian with experience in diabetes management and education should coordinate and implement MNT. All caregivers must have clear understanding of nutrition therapy and be supportive of the patient's effort to adhere to the nutrition plan.

■ Nutrition Recommendations

A personalized nutrition plan should be based on individual evaluation, taking into account factors such as biochemical parameters, physical status, social history, medical regimen, and dietary patterns and preferences. It may be necessary to modify the plan based on therapeutic outcomes or the patient's capacity to make lifestyle changes.

Nutrition recommendations for all people with diabetes are listed in the **Table 7.1**. They focus on lifestyle goals and strategies for the prevention and treatment of diabetes rather than advocating a single "standard" diet.

It should be noted that high-protein, high-fat, low-carbohydrate diets, such as The Atkins Diet, have recently attracted a great deal of attention. This type of diet revolves around the basic tenet that increased consumption of protein-rich foods (ie, red meat) and reduced intake of carbohydrates mobilize body glycogen stores, resulting in intracellular water loss. Although there is greater water loss and, hence, weight loss in the early phase of this type of diet, water equilibrium is reestablished in the second and subsequent weeks, so that weight loss becomes a function of energy deficit. If carbohydrate restriction is severe, ketosis can result, possibly leading to hyperuricemia as ketones compete with uric acid for renal tubular excretion. In general, these meat-based, low-fiber diets are not recommended for patients with type 1 diabetes because of their potential adverse effects on kidney function.

■ Strategies for Type 1 Diabetes

The following principles of MNT are fundamental to intensified management, regardless of specific meal-planning strategies:

- Base the initial meal plan on the patient's normal intake of calories, selection of food, and timing of meals.

- Select an insulin regimen consistent with the patient's usual routines of eating, sleeping, and physical activity.
- Match insulin administration to mealtimes based on the types of insulin used.
- Monitor blood glucose levels and, if necessary, adjust the basic insulin doses and regimen according to food intake.
- Monitor glycosylated hemoglobin (A1C), weight, blood pressure, lipids, and other relevant biochemical parameters and modify the meal plan to meet desired goals.

For patients practicing intensive therapy, it is essential to develop individualized algorithms for the interrelationship of insulin, carbohydrate intake, and exercise so that systematic adjustments may be made in response to deviations from normal patterns. Chapter 8, *Multiple-Component Insulin Therapy,* describes these algorithmic approaches in detail.

Exercise

Regular physical activity is recommended as an important aspect of therapy for all patients with diabetes. Exercise decreases insulin requirements in patients with type 1 diabetes and can improve cardiovascular (CV) risk factors (such as weight, blood pressure, and blood lipid levels) while enhancing a sense of well-being. In 2002, the National Academies' Institute of Medicine recommended 60 minutes of exercise per day, doubling previous recommendations. However, before increasing usual patterns of physical activity, patients with diabetes should undergo a thorough medical evaluation to screen for the presence of macrovascular and microvascular complications (see Chapter 14, *Long-term Complications*). In particular,

TABLE 7.1 — Target Nutrition Recommendations for People With Diabetes

Carbohydrate
- The total amount of carbohydrate in meals or snacks is more important than the source or type.
- Carbohydrate and monounsaturated fat should together provide 60% to 70% of energy intake. Consider the metabolic profile and need for weight loss when determining the monounsaturated fat content of the diet.
- Sucrose and sucrose-containing foods do not need to be restricted.
- Non-nutritive sweeteners are safe when consumed within the acceptable daily intake levels established by the Food and Drug Administration.
- People with diabetes need not consume a greater amount of dietary fiber than nondiabetics.
- The use of low-glycemic foods may reduce postprandial hyperglycemia; insufficient evidence of any long-term benefits of using low-glycemic index diets precludes their use as a primary strategy in food/meal planning.

Protein
- There is no evidence to suggest that usual protein intake (15% to 20% of total daily energy) should be modified if renal function is normal.
- In individuals with microalbuminuria, reduction of protein to 0.8-1.0 g/kg body weight/day, and in individuals with overt nephropathy, reduction to 0.8 g/kg body weight/day, may slow the progression of nephropathy.
- The long-term effects of diets high in protein and low in carbohydrate are unknown and may have specific renal and cardiovascular risks.

Fat
- <10% of energy intake should be derived from saturated fats. Those with low-density lipoprotein (LDL) cholesterol $\geq$100 mg/dL may benefit from lowering saturated fat intake to <7% of energy intake.

Continued

- Dietary cholesterol intake should be <300 mg/day. Those with LDL cholesterol ≥100 mg/dL may benefit from lowering dietary cholesterol to <200 mg/day.
- Minimize intake of transunsaturated fatty acids.
- Approximately 10% of energy intake should be derived from polyunsaturated fats.

Micronutrients
- There is no clear evidence of benefit from vitamin or mineral supplementation, including antioxidants, in people with diabetes who do not have underlying deficiencies. Exceptions include folate for prevention of birth defects and calcium for prevention of bone disease.

Alcohol
- Daily intake should be limited to 1 drink for adult women and 2 drinks for adult men. One drink is defined as 12 oz beer, 5 oz wine, or 1.5 oz approximately 80 proof spirits.
- To reduce risk of hypoglycemia, alcohol should be consumed with food.

Sodium
- Reduction in sodium intake lowers blood pressure.
- The goal is sodium intake of ≤2,400 mg (≤100 mmol)/day.

Adapted from: Klingensmith GJ, ed. *Intensive Diabetes Management*. 3rd ed. Alexandria, Va: American Diabetes Association; 2003:140.

a graded exercise test may be helpful if a patient, about to begin a moderate- to high-intensity physical activity program, is at high risk for underlying CV disease according to one of the following criteria:

- Age >35 years
- Age >25 years and
  - Type 2 diabetes >10 years' duration
  - Type 1 diabetes >15 years' duration
- Presence of any additional risk factor for coronary artery disease

- Presence of microvascular disease
- Peripheral vascular disease
- Autonomic neuropathy.

In patients with nonspecific electrocardiogram changes, a radionuclide stress test should be considered. In those planning to participate in low-intensity forms of exercise (<60% of maximal heart rate), clinical judgment is required to decide if an exercise stress test is required.

■ Preparing for Exercise

Several precautionary measures should be taken by people with diabetes in preparation for exercise. Protecting the feet is essential, particularly for individuals with peripheral neuropathy. The use of silica gel or air midsoles as well as polyester or blend (cotton/polyester) socks to prevent blisters and keep the feet dry is important for minimizing foot trauma. Additionally, special precautions must be taken to avoid hypoglycemia. These measures include:

- Wearing a medical ID bracelet or other medical identification
- Being alert to symptoms of hypoglycemia
- Measuring blood glucose before exercise to ensure that the level exceeds 100 mg/dL
- Carrying a form of quick-acting carbohydrate to treat hypoglycemia should it occur
- Teaching family members and friends about glucagon therapy
- Learning glycemic response to different physical activity conditions.

Because physical activity may further increase blood glucose levels in patients with poorly controlled diabetes, exercise should be avoided if fasting glucose levels are >250 mg/dL and ketosis is present, and caution should be observed if glucose levels are >300 mg/

dL and no ketosis is present. The advice of an exercise physiologist can be helpful in devising a successful exercise program.

SUGGESTED READING

Franz MJ, Bantle JP, Beebe CA, et al. Evidence-based nutrition principles and recommendations for the treatment and prevention of diabetes and related complications. *Diabetes Care*. 2003; 26(suppl 1):S51-S61.

Klingensmith GJ, ed. *Intensive Diabetes Management*. 3rd ed. Alexandria, Va: American Diabetes Association; 2003.

Ruderman N, Devlin JT, eds. *The Health Professional's Guide to Diabetes and Exercise*. Alexandria, Va: American Diabetes Association; 1995.

Zinman B, Ruderman N, Campaigne BN, Devlin JT, Schneider SH, American Diabetes Association. Physical activity/exercise and diabetes mellitus. *Diabetes Care*. 2003;26(suppl 1):S73-S77.

7

8

Multiple-Component Insulin Therapy

Contemporary management of type 1 diabetes is founded on the premise that maintaining glycosylated hemoglobin (A1C) levels <7% reduces the incidence and progression of neuropathy, nephropathy, and retinopathy, as demonstrated by the Diabetes Control and Complications Trial. The aim of therapy has thus moved beyond extending the duration of life to improving the quality of life through stringent glycemic control. Integral to this shift has been the development of insulin analogues that, compared with standard insulins such as regular and neutral protamine Hagedorn (NPH), make intensive diabetes management involving multiple–daily-injection regimens more convenient, safe, and effective. Because the onset and duration of action of these novel insulins resemble human insulin secretion more closely than those of older preparations, basal and prandial insulin may be replaced separately, thus simplifying insulin dosing and adjustment, increasing flexibility, and reducing the risk of hypoglycemia.

This chapter describes practical approaches to multiple-component insulin therapy, including discussions of:

- Physiologic vs nonphysiologic models of insulin replacement
- Available insulin products
- Factors influencing insulin absorption
- Specific multicomponent regimens
- Insulin doses and adjustments.

Physiologic vs Nonphysiologic Insulin Replacement

Insulin replacement regimens are defined largely by the pharmacokinetic and pharmacodynamic profiles of available insulin products (**Table 8.1**). Until relatively recently, one of the major obstacles to achieving target glycemia (A1C <7%) in patients with type 1 diabetes was the inability to replicate normal patterns of insulin secretion given the time-action profiles of conventional subcutaneously injected insulin formulations. Physicians' concerns about the complexity of maintaining stringent glycemic control with these insulins and the need to avoid hypoglycemia resulted in the use of *nonphysiologic insulin replacement* strategies that did not attempt to mimic normal β-cell secretion (**Figure 8.1**). Although these nonphysiologic strategies, consisting of once- or twice-daily basal injections, are sometimes adequate for newly diagnosed patients with type 1 diabetes or those with latent autoimmune diabetes of adults (LADA) who are still producing endogenous insulin, they are not considered appropriate for patients who are severely insulin deficient.

Programs of physiologic insulin replacement, by contrast, aim to mimic normal insulin secretion by addressing basal and prandial insulin needs (**Figure 8.2**). In these regimens, basal (or background) insulin is used to suppress hepatic glucose production when food is not eaten (ie, overnight and between meals after food absorption, when a relatively flat insulin concentration is required); prandial (or bolus) insulin is used to control glycemia associated with meals (when a sharp increase in plasma insulin is needed to facilitate glucose disposal at the muscle).

Up-to-date management of type 1 diabetes attempts to emulate these two components of normal insulin secretion to safely achieve and maintain near-normal glycemia (A1C <7%). Yet the time-action profiles of standard insulins can impede this effort because they do not readily allow for the clear separation of basal and prandial insulin action. For example, the classic twice-daily "split-mixed" regimen of NPH and regular insulin, although considered physiologic, uses each insulin component to meet both prandial and basal needs (**Figure 8.3**). Although the regular insulin is responsible for peripheral glucose disposal at breakfast and dinner, its effective duration (approximately 3 to 6 hours) frequently extends through lunch, making it a prandial insulin for that meal as well. At the same time, the NPH insulin, with an effective duration of 10 to 16 hours, functions as a basal insulin after absorption of breakfast and lunch, but because of its relatively rapid onset, also serves as part of the prandial insulin component at breakfast and as the primary prandial insulin at lunch. Compensating for the inherent variability of this overlapping action requires strict and consistent coordination as to the timing of injections and meals, especially in patients aiming for stringent glycemic control for whom delaying lunch or skipping a midmorning snack may result in hypoglycemia.

A simpler conceptual approach preferred by many patients with diabetes is using a prandial insulin for each meal (ie, regular insulin, insulin lispro, aspart, or glulisine) and a separate basal insulin (ie, NPH, insulin zinc susptension [Lente], extended insulin zinc susptension [Ultralente], insulin glargine [Lantus], or, pending approval by the Food and Drug Administration [FDA], basal insulin detemir) (**Figure 8.4**). Although these true basal-prandial regimens require more shots than conventional twice-daily regimens, they are considerably more flexible, allowing greater freedom to skip meals or change mealtimes. Moreover, use of the 24-hour basal insulin analogue, insulin glargine, and the rapid-acting insulin analogues, insulins lispro,

TABLE 8.1 — Currently Available Insulin Preparations

Insulin Preparation*	Onset of Action (h)	Peak Action (h)	Effective duration of Action (h)	Maximum Duration (h)
Rapid-acting analogues				
Insulin lispro (Humalog)	5–15 min	½ – 1½	5	4–6
Insulin aspart (NovoLog)	5–15 min	½ – 1½	5	4–6
Insulin glulisine (Apidra)	5–15 min	½ – 1½	5	4–6
Short-acting				
Regular (soluble)	½ – 1	2–3	5–8	6–10
Intermediate-acting				
NPH (isophane)	2–4	4–10	10–16	14–18
Lente (insulin zinc suspension)	2–4	4–12	12–18	16–20
Long-acting				
Ultralente (extended insulin zinc suspension)	6–10	10–16	18–24	20–24

Long-acting analogue				
Insulin glargine (Lantus)	2–4†	No peak	20–24	24
Combinations				
70/30 (70% NPH, 30% regular)	½ – 1	Dual	10–16	14–18
50/50 (50% NPH, 50% regular)	½ – 1	Dual	10–16	14–18
Combination analogues				
75/25 (75% NPL, 25% insulin lispro)	5–15 min	Dual	10–16	14–18
70/30 (70% NPL, 30% insulin aspart)	5–15 min	Dual	10–16	14–18

Abbreviations: NPL, neutral protamine lispro; NPH, neutral protamine Hagedorn.

* Assuming 0.1–0.2 U/kg per injection; onset and duration vary significantly by injection site.
† Time to steady state

Adapted from: Hirsch IB, Trence DL. *Optimizing Diabetes Care for the Practitioner*. Philadelphia, Pa: Lippincott Williams and Wilkins; 2003:38 and DeWitt DE, Hirsch IB. *JAMA*. 2003;289:2255.

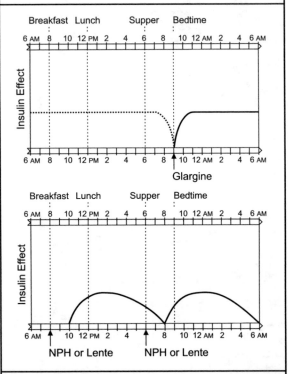

FIGURE 8.1 — Examples of Nonphysiologic Insulin Replacement

Top: Nonphysiologic insulin replacement does not mimic normal β-cell secretion. These regimens are not recommended for patients with type 1 diabetes. A once-daily, long-acting insulin glargine is released with a relatively flat delivery of approximately 20 to 24 hours in most patients. Dashed line indicates the effective duration of glargine continuing through the following day. *Bottom:* Twice-daily, intermediate-acting neutral protamine Hagedorn (isophane insulin; NPH) and Lente (insulin zinc) are commonly used as basal insulin. Arrows indicate insulin injection.

DeWitt DE, Hirsch IB. *JAMA*. 2003;289:2257.

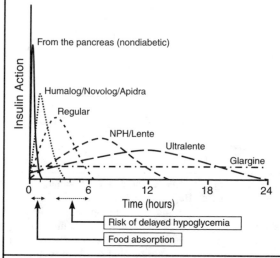

FIGURE 8.2 — Peak Action of Insulin Compared With Peak Rise in Glucose After Eating

From the pancreas (nondiabetic)

Humalog/Novolog/Apidra

Regular

NPH/Lente

Ultralente

Glargine

Insulin Action

Time (hours)

0   6   12   18   24

Risk of delayed hypoglycemia

Food absorption

The time course of action (pharmacokinetics) for the fast-acting insulin analogs *(dotted line)* is not as fast as insulin from the pancreas of a nondiabetic individual *(solid line),* but it is much more physiologic than the older regular insulin preparations *(short-dashed line).* Also shown is the time course of action of the intermediate- and long-acting insulins, including the new long-acting insulin analogue glargine (Lantus).

aspart, and glulisine, makes altering strategies to achieve individually defined blood glucose targets easier. Such modifications might include changing the timing of insulin injections in relation to meals, changing the portions or content of food to be consumed, or adjusting insulin doses or supplements.

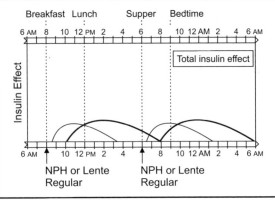

FIGURE 8.3 — Example of Conventional Physiologic Insulin Regimen

Physiologic insulin replacement with intermediate-acting neutral protamine Hagedorn (isophane insulin; NPH) or Lente (insulin zinc) and short-acting regular insulin (shown in a ratio of 70:30) attempts to mimic normal β-cell secretion. Each insulin serves as both a basal and a prandial insulin. Meal timing and consistency are important for patients using this regimen. Many patients require a midmorning and bedtime snack to prevent hypoglycemia when the effect of the two insulins overlap at late morning and nighttime. Moving the dinnertime NPH injection to bedtime decreases the risk of nocturnal hypoglycemia. Arrows indicate insulin injection.

DeWitt DE, Hirsch IB. *JAMA.* 2003;289:2257.

Selecting an Insulin Preparation

■ Types of Insulin

Selecting the appropriate insulin depends largely on the desired time course of insulin action. **Table 8.1** shows the pharmacokinetic characteristics—time to onset of action, time of peak action, effective duration of action, and maximum duration of action—of currently available insulins; however, these can vary considerably among individuals.

Insulin products are categorized according to their action profiles:

- Rapid-acting: eg, insulin lispro, aspart, and glulisine (genetically engineered insulin analogues)
- Short-acting: eg, regular (soluble) insulin
- Intermediate-acting: eg, NPH or Lente
- Long-acting: eg, Ultralente, insulin glargine, and, pending FDA approval, insulin detemir (genetically engineered insulin analogues).

A general principle to bear in mind is the longer the time to peak, the broader the peak and the longer the duration of action. Additionally, the breadth of the peak and the duration of action will be extended somewhat with increasing dose.

Rapid-Acting Insulin

The genetically engineered insulin analogues insulin lispro, aspart, and glulisine, have a rapid onset of 15 to 30 minutes, a peak in 30 to 90 minutes, and have an effective duration of 3 to 4 hours when injected subcutaneously because they do not self-aggregate in solution as human (regular) insulin does. Insulin lispro differs from human insulin by an amino acid exchange of lysine and proline at positions 28 and 29. The substitution of aspartic acid for proline at position 28 characterizes insulin aspart. Insulin glulisine was developed by replacing the asparagine in position B3 by lysine, and lysine at position B29 by glutamic acid. Rapid-acting insulins are most suitably used at mealtime as prandial insulin or in insulin pumps.

Short-Acting Insulin

Regular insulin has a delay to onset of action of 30 to 60 minutes, a peak of 2 to 3 hours, and an effective duration of 3 to 6 hours. Proper use requires injection 20 to 30 minutes prior to meals to match insulin

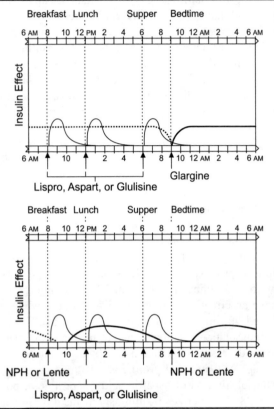

FIGURE 8.4 — Examples of Physiologic Insulin Delivery Regimen

Top: Once-daily glargine with lispro, aspart, or glulisine (shown in a ratio of 50:50) allows patients to skip meals or change mealtimes. Insulins lispro, aspart, and glulisine (rapid-acting) are prandial insulins and glargine (long-acting) is a basal insulin. This regimen is easier to use since it features true basal and prandial insulins. Dashed line indicates the effective duration of glargine continuing through the following day. Glargine achieves steady state at approximately 2 hours. *Bottom:* Intermediate-act-

Continued

ing neutral protamine Hagedorn (isophane insulin; NPH) and Lente (insulin zinc) are basal insulins. Rapid-acting lispro, aspart, and glulisine insulins are prandial insulins. This regimen (shown in a ratio of 50:50) is more difficult to adjust because NPH can act as both a basal and a prandial insulin. Dashed line indicates the effective duration of NPH or Lente continuing through the following day. Arrows indicate insulin injection.

DeWitt DE, Hirsch IB. *JAMA*. 2003;289:2258.

availability and carbohydrate absorption. Regular insulin acts almost instantly when injected intravenously.

Intermediate-Acting Insulin

NPH insulin is slowly absorbed due to the addition of protamine to regular insulin. Its onset of action occurs 2 to 4 hours from the time of injection, with a peak effect lasting 6 to 10 hours, and an effective duration of 10 to 16 hours. Lente insulin, which is regular insulin bound to zinc, has a slightly longer effective duration than NPH. It is important to note that regular insulin may bind with Lente or Ultralente, which blunts its effect. Therefore, whenever regular insulin is mixed with these agents, it should be injected immediately. The mix should not be left in the syringe for any length of time. Lente and NPH are commonly used as twice-daily basal insulins.

Long-Acting Insulin

Ultralente insulin is absorbed slowly in its zinc crystalline form, with an onset of action occurring 6 to 10 hours from the time of injection, a peak effect of 10 to 16 hours, and an effective duration of 18 to 20 hours. When mixed with regular insulin, it must be injected immediately. Insulin glargine, a modified human insulin that forms a microprecipitate in the subcutaneous (SC) tissue, is released slowly with no pronounced peak over the course of about 20 to 24

79

hours in most patients. Insulin detemir is a soluble basal insulin analogue which is under development. It is covalently acylated with fatty acids on lysine at position 29, which enhances its binding to albumin and thus retards its absorption from SC tissue.

Insulin Mixtures

Premixed preparations of regular and NPH insulins, insulin lispro protamine suspension (NPL) and insulin lispro, and insulin aspart protamine suspension (NPA) and insulin aspart are commercially available. Although these products may be helpful for elderly patients, blind patients, or others who cannot easily mix insulin in the syringe, they limit flexibility and are not useful for patients involved in intensive insulin programs.

Factors Influencing Insulin Absorption

Insulin absorption variability is the greatest obstacle to replicating physiologic insulin secretion. Among the many factors that affect insulin absorption and availability (**Table 8.2**) are injection site, the timing, type or dose of insulin used, and physical activity. Day-to-day intraindividual variation in insulin absorption is approximately 25%, and the variation between patients may be as high as 50%. One reason for this is that large doses of human insulin form an insulin depot, which can unpredictably prolong duration of action; this is less of an issue with insulin analogues, however. Thus patients injecting 40 U of NPH insulin into their abdomen before breakfast, for example, may have a markedly different onset and peak of action than the same patients injecting 20 U of NPH into their thigh in the evening; mixing insulin lispro with the morning NPH dose and regular insulin with the evening dose would also lead to further variation, especially if the NPH is not resuspended properly. In

TABLE 8.2 — Factors Affecting the Bioavailability and Absorption Rate of Subcutaneously Injected Insulin

Factor	Effects
Site of injection	Abdominal injection (particularly if above the umbilicus) results in the quickest absorption; arm injection results in quicker absorption than thigh or hip injection.
Depth of injection	Intramuscular injections are absorbed more rapidly than subcutaneous injections.
Insulin concentration	U-40 insulin (40 U/mL) is absorbed more rapid than U-100 insulin (100 U/mL).
Insulin dose	Higher doses have prolonged durations of action compared with lower doses.
Insulin mixing	Regular insulin maintains its potency and time-action profile when it is mixed with NPH insulin; however, mixing regular insulin with Lente or Ultralente insulin slows absorption and blunts the activity of regular insulin.
Exercise	Exercising a muscle group before injecting insulin into that area increases the rate of insulin absorption.
Heat application or massage	Local application of heat or massage after an insulin injection increases the rate of insulin absorption.

Hirsch IB. *Am Fam Physician*. 1999; 60:2343-2356.

8

general, any strategy that increases the consistency of delivery should decrease glucose fluctuations; and insulin regimens that emphasize shorter-acting insulins are more reproducible in their effects on blood glucose levels.

Insulin pens are convenient and their use may avert some insulin errors, but insulin cartridges for pens are more costly than insulin in vials. Insulin pumps using only regular insulin or rapid-acting insulin analogues significantly reduce variability. Like multiple-injection regimens, use of an insulin pump requires frequent blood glucose monitoring, as well as a backup method of insulin administration and attention to mechanical and injection site issues.

■ Reducing Absorption Variability
Injection Site
Insulin is absorbed most rapidly when injected into the abdomen, followed by the arm, buttocks, and thigh. These regional differences in absorption rate, which are likely caused by variations in blood flow, are significant when using conventional insulin preparations such as regular and NPH; thus with these agents in particular, the practice of rotating injection sites between regions should be avoided. Alternatively, rotating injection sites within the same region for any given injection will result in more predictable day-to-day blood glucose control.

In some situations, it is possible to take advantage of regional differences in absorption to suit a patient's individual insulin needs. For example, because insulin is absorbed fastest in the abdomen, some patients use the abdomen for preprandial injections of regular insulin. Or, if an intermediate-acting insulin is used to provide basal insulin for a significant portion of the day ($\geq$15 hours), it may be desirable to inject into a site from which absorption is slow, ie, the thigh. When the duration of action is longer or shorter than desired, a site may be chosen with faster or slower absorption.

Timing of Premeal Injections

Gauging the appropriate interval between preprandial injections and eating, known as the "lag time," is essential for coordinating insulin availability with glycemic excursions following meals. The timing of the injections should also be adapted to the level of premeal glycemia. Insulins lispro, aspart, and glulisine have rapid onset of action and, ideally, should be given approximately 10 minutes before mealtime when blood glucose is in the target range; however, provided there is no hyperglycemia or hypoglycemia present, either agent may be administered within 10 minutes of meal consumption or immediately prior to eating if preferred. Regular insulin administered subcutaneously is best administered at least 20 to 30 minutes before eating if blood glucose levels are within target, keeping in mind that if the meal is delayed, hypoglycemia may ensue. When blood glucose levels are above a patient's target range, the lag time should be increased to permit the insulin to begin to have an effect sooner. In this case, rapid-acting insulin analogues can be given 15 minutes and regular insulin 30 to 60 minutes before the meal. If premeal blood glucose levels are below target range, administration of regular insulin should be delayed until immediately before eating, and injections of rapid-acting insulin should be postponed until after some carbohydrates have been consumed.

Other Factors Influencing Insulin Absorption

Physical activity increases blood flow to the area under exertion and therefore accelerates absorption of insulin from that region. Whenever possible, patients should avoid injecting in such areas while insulin is being absorbed. For example, if a patient intends to do sit-ups after insulin administration, it is best to avoid injecting in the abdomen. However, the abdomen is preferable to the thigh if the planned exercise is jogging. Other factors influencing absorption of regular insulin are ambient temperature, smoking, and direct massage of the injection site. Also, thin patients with little SC tissue may absorb insulin more rapidly because the injections may in fact be intramuscular. In this case, it could be beneficial to switch to insulin formulations that are absorbed more slowly, eg, using regular insulin instead of preprandial insulin lispro.

Role of Insulin Analogues

Most of the problems of insulin replacement in type 1 diabetes arise from the fact that SC injection or infusion remains the most common route of administration. From the SC site of injection, insulin is absorbed into the systemic not the portal circulation. More importantly, SC injection leads to variable absorption from one injection to another, due largely to the nonphysiologic pharmacokinetics of standard insulins. Insulin analogues were developed to overcome this problem.

Three rapid-acting analogues, lispro, aspart, and glulisine, are currently approved for use in the United States. Although the primary structure of these three insulins differ, practically speaking these three preparations exhibit the same pharmacokinetics and dynamics after SC injection, closely mimicking normal postprandial insulin response. All three have a rapid onset of action (15 to 30 minutes), peak in 30 to 90 minutes, and have a duration of action of approximately 3 hours, thereby improving 1- to 2-hour postprandial blood glucose control compared with regular insulin. They offer the advantage of greater flexibility because patients can inject immediately before eating and thus better match their dose of insulin to calorie and carbohydrate intake. However, these rapid-acting analogues must be used in conjunction with a basal insulin to improve overall glycemic control.

Basal insulin glargine is a once-daily, 20- to 24-hour human insulin analogue distinguished from native human insulin by alterations in both the A and B chains. The resulting molecule has its isoelectric point shifted form a pH of 5.4 to 6.7, making it more soluble at a slightly acidic pH and less soluble at the physiologic pH of SC tissue. When injected subcutaneously, glargine forms a microprecipitate at the physiologic pH of the SC tissue. Slow dissolution of the glargine precipitate at the injection site results in relatively constant release, with no pronounced peak over 24 hours, providing a basal insulin supply comparable to that of healthy individuals. The clear solution does not require resuspension (usually by rolling the vial or cartridge) before injection, eliminating a major source of variability characteristic of insoluble suspensions such as NPH insulin and Ultralente insulin. However, this property also prohibits the mixing of glargine with other insulins.

Clinical trials have demonstrated lower fasting glucose levels and less nocturnal hypoglycemia with insulin glargine than with NPH, advantages that are especially relevant in patients aiming for meticulous control (A1C <7%) or those with hypoglycemia unawareness.

Another promising long-acting insulin analogue, detemir, is under development. Detemir is covalently acylated with fatty acids on lysine at position 29, which increases its binding to albumin and thus delays its absorption from SC tissue. In patients with type 1 diabetes, detemir and NPH proved to be equally effective in maintaining glycemic control, although detemir was administered at a higher molar dose.

Patients with type 1 diabetes derive the greatest therapeutic benefit when basal and prandial analogues are used together, because the physiologic pharmacokinetics and pharmacodynamics of these analogues make separating the basal and prandial components of insulin replacement easier. As a general rule of thumb, half the insulin is used as a basal insulin, while the other half is used as a prandial insulin. The amount of prandial insulin can initially be determined by approximating the amount of calories consumed at each meal. As patients become more educated, however, they may alter the prandial dose by estimating the carbohydrate component of each meal or snack.

Multiple-Component Insulin Regimens

Patients with type 1 diabetes who have no endogenous insulin secretion require multiple components of insulin replacement that replicate the prandial and basal action of physiologic insulin secretion. Thus mealtime, between-meal, and overnight insulin needs must be determined and action taken in response to self-monitoring of blood glucose (SMBG) levels or an unusual situation that can affect glycemia. The most flexible regimens for stringent glycemic control:

- Stress the need for preprandial insulin before each meal, apart from basal insulin
- Allow ample choice with respect to the size and timing of meals, plus the potential for omitting meals while still balancing food consumption with physical activity and insulin dosage
- Include frequent monitoring of therapy to facilitate full participation in the experiences of normal life.

A key aspect of any flexible program is frequent SMBG, ie, at least 4 times daily. The results are used to help patients make appropriate changes in insulin dosage and timing, carbohydrate intake, and physical activity. The changes are made according to a predetermined action plan provided to the patient by the health care team. This plan consists of an individualized set of algorithms and should be clearly distinguished from sliding-scale insulin therapy, which is an outdated approach that entails retrospective correction of hyperglycemia with short-acting insulin regardless of caloric intake or the considerations of physiologic insulin delivery.

■ Prandial Insulin Therapy

Physiologic prandial insulin secretion is best replaced by giving preprandial injections of a rapid-acting insulin analogue (lispro, aspart, or glulisine) before each meal by syringe, pen, or pump. Each preprandial insulin dose is individually adjusted, taking into account the current blood glucose and the carbohydrate content of the meal. In a flexible plan, the timing of meals need not be rigidly scheduled and meals can be skipped along with the accompanying prandial insulin dose.

Regular insulin is another option for prandial glycemic control. It is not as convenient as the insulin analogues, however, because of its longer time to onset and peak effect. Therefore, injection at least 20 to 30 minutes (or longer) before a given meal is required to coordinate its action with meal-related glycemic excursions.

The practice of mixing rapid-acting analogues and regular insulin together, referred to as an "insulin cocktail," became popular when lispro was first introduced. The lispro accelerated the onset of the prandial insulin coverage, while the extended action of the regular insulin made up for the inadequate basal insulin coverage by NPH or Lente insulin. Although the proportion varied, it often started with 50% of each insulin administered before mealtimes, with the intermediate-acting NPH or Lente insulin injected at bedtime. In general, the regular insulin was a fixed dose at each meal, while the lispro varied according to carbohydrate intake and the current blood glucose level.

Over the past few years, insulin cocktails have been supplanted by the use of a rapid-acting prandial insulin (lispro, aspart, or glulisine) and basal insulin glargine. The improved basal coverage of once-daily, 24-hour insulin glargine compared with NPH negates the need for the regular insulin at mealtime.

■ Basal Insulin Therapy

Basal insulin is administered in one of three ways:

- An intermediate-acting insulin (NPH) at bedtime and as a small morning dose
- One or two daily injections of long-acting insulin (Ultralente or glargine)
- The basal component of a continuous subcutaneous insulin infusion (CSII) program.

It should be noted that with a clearly differentiated basal insulin component (eg, glargine or pump therapy), patients need approximately half of their insulin as basal insulin. When beginning a basal-prandial regimen, patients should decrease the calculated 50% basal insulin dosing by 20% to avoid hypoglycemia. Using this calculation, one third of patients will be receiving the correct dose, one third will need more, and one third will need less basal insulin.

The advantages of insulin glargine over NPH were demonstrated in a recent study comparing the efficacy of these agents in patients with type 1 diabetes using insulin lispro at mealtimes. Compared with subjects using NPH four times daily, patients using once-daily glargine either at dinnertime or bedtime had:

- Lower fasting, premeal, and postmeal blood glucose results (**Figure 8.5**)
- A greater percentage of glucose values in the target range, primarily in the fasting state, before meals, and at night

- A greater reduction in A1C
- A lower frequency of hypoglycemia, especially at night
- Less variability of blood glucose at night.

Additionally, the time of evening administration of insulin glargine (ie, dinnertime vs bedtime) did not affect blood glucose levels. Thus whereas NPH should ideally be given at bedtime to curb the frequency of nocturnal hypoglycemia, insulin glargine can be injected either at dinnertime or bedtime without compromising glycemic control.

FIGURE 8.5 — Daily Blood Glucose in Three Groups of Patients With Type 1 Diabetes

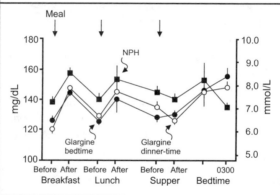

Daily blood glucose (data from blood glucose monitoring of the last month of 3-month study) in three groups of patients with type 1 diabetes on intensive insulin treatment and lispro insulin at mealtime, given basal insulin either as NPH 4 times/day or insulin glargine once daily at dinnertime or bedtime.

Rossetti P, et al. *Diabetes Care*. 2003;26:1492.

Specific Flexible Insulin Therapy Regimens

■ Rapid-Acting Prandial and Intermediate-Acting Basal Insulin

This regimen uses a rapid-acting insulin injection (lispro, aspart, or glulisine) before each meal and an intermediate-acting insulin (NPH) given at bedtime to cover overnight insulin needs as well as the increased insulin requirements that occur before breakfast, known as the "dawn phenomenon" (**Figure 8.6**). With this approach, serum insulin levels before breakfast are higher (better matching insulin needs) and nocturnal hypoglycemia is less of a problem. A small morning dose of NPH insulin (perhaps 20% to 30% of the bedtime dose) is often enough to address daytime basal insulin needs, although it may also be necessary to include some NPH insulin prior to dinner and/or lunch if the interval between breakfast and dinner or dinner and bedtime is prolonged and the effects of the morning NPH insulin have worn off.

This popular insulin regimen is relatively easy to understand and allows flexibility in the size and timing of meals. Because each meal corresponds with a distinct insulin component providing primary insulin action, doses of rapid-acting insulin may be adjusted as required.

■ Rapid-Acting Insulin and Long-Acting Basal Insulin

In this regimen, long-acting basal insulin glargine (**Figure 8.7**) or basal Ultralente insulin (**Figure 8.8**) is used with three preprandial injections of insulin lispro, aspart, and glulisine. The insulin analogue glargine has a broad peak 8 to 16 hours after injection and a sustained action of 20 to 24 hours. Clinically, glargine acts as a peakless insulin, reducing episodes of hypoglycemia, especially at night. How-

FIGURE 8.6 — Schematic Representation of Idealized Insulin Effect Provided by Multiple-Dose Regimens Featuring Basal Intermediate-Acting Insulin

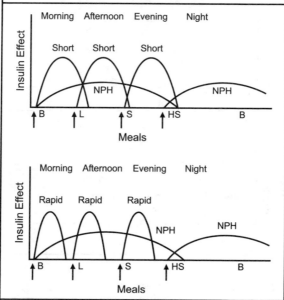

Abbreviations: B, breakfast; HS, bedtime; L, lunch; NPH, neutral protamine Hagedorn [insulin]; S, supper.

Schematic representation of idealized insulin effect provided by multiple-dose regimens featuring basal intermediate-acting insulin at bedtime and before breakfast and preprandial injections of short- (*top*) or rapid- (*bottom*) acting insulin. Arrows indicate time of insulin injection.

Klingensmith G, ed, for the American Diabetes Association. *Intensive Diabetes Management*. 3rd ed. New York, NY: The McGraw-Hill Companies; 2003:83.

FIGURE 8.7 — Schematic Representation of Idealized Insulin Effect Provided by Multiple-Dose Regimens Featuring Basal Long-Acting Insulin Glargine

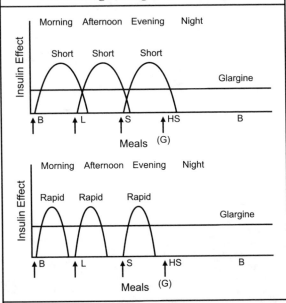

Abbreviations: B, breakfast; G, glargine; HS, bedtime; L, lunch; S, dinner.

Schematic representation of idealized insulin effect provided by multiple-dose regimen featuring basal long-acting insulin glargine and preprandial injections of short- (*top*) or rapid- (*bottom*) acting insulin. Arrows indicate time of insulin injection.

Klingensmith G, ed, for the American Diabetes Association. *Intensive Diabetes Management*. 3rd ed. New York, NY: The McGraw-Hill Companies; 2003:84.

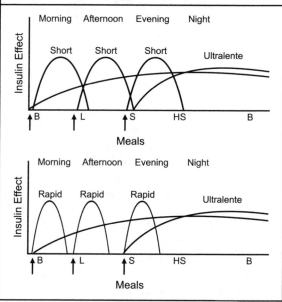

FIGURE 8.8 — Schematic Representation of Idealized Insulin Effect Provided by Multiple-Dose Regimens Featuring Long-Acting Ultralente Insulin

Abbreviations: B, breakfast; HS, bedtime; L, lunch; S, supper.

Schematic representation of idealized insulin effect provided by multiple-dose regimen featuring long-acting Ultralente insulin and preprandial injections of short- (*top*) or rapid- (*bottom*) acting insulin. Arrows indicate time of insulin injection.

Klingensmith G, ed, for the American Diabetes Association. *Intensive Diabetes Management*. 3rd ed. New York, NY: The McGraw-Hill Companies; 2003:85.

ever, if used at dinnertime, the waning that occurs at 18 to 24 hours could lead to late afternoon hyperglycemia. Hence, a once-daily bedtime injection of glargine may provide better coverage. Recent findings indicate that it is safe to use insulin glargine any time of the day, as long as it is the same time each day. For young children, who require little basal insulin between 4 AM and 7 AM, morning administration may be best.

Human Ultralente insulin has a broad peak of approximately 10 to 16 hours after administration and may have sustained action up to 24 hours, although its absorption is variable. It is easiest to start Ultralente insulin at approximately 50% of the total daily dose, with one half of the dose administered with breakfast and the remainder with the evening meal.

Persistent fasting hyperglycemia may be treated by increasing the dose of Ultralente insulin given at the evening meal. However, in some patients, this approach leads to nocturnal hypoglycemia without any improvement in fasting hyperglycemia owing to the dawn phenomenon. A reasonable alternative is administering Ultralente in the morning and NPH as the other basal component at bedtime. The benefit of this regimen is that early-morning insulin resistance is targeted with the bedtime NPH insulin. In thin patients who appear to absorb human insulin (both Ultralente and intermediate-acting insulin) more quickly, it may be advisable to use human Ultralente as if it were an intermediate-acting insulin.

Continuous Subcutaneous Insulin Infusion

CSII with an insulin pump will be discussed at length in Chapter 9, *Continuous Subcutaneous Insulin Infusion*. This is an especially accurate way to deliver insulin and is considered the gold standard.

Pumps deliver either regular insulin or insulin lispro/aspart/glulisine at a preprogrammed basal rate. Most pumps allow patients to modulate basal rates throughout the day to correspond to the body's diurnal variations in insulin sensitivity, which would otherwise result in nighttime hypoglycemia and morning hyperglycemia. Insulin delivery can be completely suspended during a period of intense physical activity in order to avoid hypoglycemia. Additionally, a bolus of a rapid-acting analogue may be delivered immediately before a meal (or regular insulin 20 to 30 minutes before a meal) and adjusted according to the amount of carbohydrates consumed.

CSII should be considered in the following circumstances:

- When patients are motivated to improve glycemic control, especially if multiple daily injections have proven to be inadequate
- Extreme insulin sensitivity
- Need for increased flexibility with mealtimes
- Pregnancy
- Severe early morning insulin resistance (dawn phenomenon)
- Hypoglycemia unawareness.

However, CSII is not for everyone, and the decision to use a pump should be carefully considered. The best candidates for CSII:

- Appreciate the factors affecting blood glucose levels and the value of frequent blood glucose monitoring
- Have realistic expectations of CSII (eg, they understand that the pump will not manage their diabetes for them)
- Are comfortable with programmable mechanical devices
- Have stable personality traits.

Patients contemplating CSII must be instructed by a health care team experienced in the use of pumps. For more information on CSII, see Chapter 9, *Continuous Subcutaneous Insulin Infusion*.

Other Insulin Regimens

Although multiple-injection regimens that separately address basal and prandial insulin needs allow for greater flexibility and usually lead to improved glycemic control, this is not always the case: lack of motivation, education, or willingness to practice frequent monitoring of blood glucose may prompt some patients to opt for nonphysiologic regimens. Indeed, recent data indicate that 41% patients with type 1 diabetes inject insulin only once or twice per day, which is less than optimal. If patients maintain relatively consistent habits of eating and physical activity, however, and stringent glycemic control is not a priority, the regimens described below may be sufficient to meet their daily needs.

■ A Twice-Daily "Split-Mixed" Regimen

This regimen uses twice-daily administration of mixtures of regular insulin or a rapid-acting insulin analogue and NPH (**Figure 8.9**). It continues to be popular because it entails only two daily injections and is often taught to medical students in lieu of more physiologic approaches reflecting state-of-the-art practice. Unfortunately, this classic split-mixed regimen seldom achieves the American Diabetes Association's goals of therapy in type 1 diabetes.

One drawback is that the NPH insulin administered before breakfast to provide both daytime basal and lunchtime prandial insulin has a broad peak. Therefore, lunch and dinner must be eaten on time to prevent hypoglycemia, and the size of lunch cannot be changed. A more serious problem is associated with

FIGURE 8.9 — Schematic Representation of Idealized Insulin Effect Provided by a "Split-Mixed" Insulin Regimen

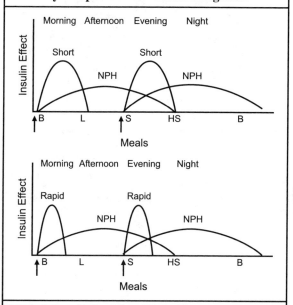

Abbreviations: B, breakfast; HS, bedtime; L, lunch; NPH, neutral protamine Hagedorn [insulin]; S, supper.

Schematic representation of idealized insulin effect provided by a split-mixed insulin regimen consisting of two daily injections of intermediate-acting insulin (NPH) and short- (*top*) or rapid- (*bottom*) acting insulin. This regimen is not recommended for patients with type 1 diabetes. Arrows indicate time of insulin injection.

Klingensmith G, ed, for the American Diabetes Association. *Intensive Diabetes Management*. 3rd ed. New York, NY: The McGraw-Hill Companies; 2003:88.

the dinnertime NPH, which produces a peak effect approximately 6 to 10 hours after injection when post-absorptive insulin needs are normally low, thereby increasing the potential for nocturnal hypoglycemia. Additionally, the effects of NPH begin to subside toward dawn when insulin resistance increases along with insulin requirements. This can lead to morning hyperglycemia, especially if the patient experiences a strong dawn phenomenon. Attempts to correct this hyperglycemia by increasing the dose of insulin, especially in the case of regular insulin, can further magnify the risk for hypoglycemia, creating a cycle of glycemic instability.

■ Split-Mixed Regimen With Bedtime NPH

This regimen consists of a mixture of regular or rapid-acting insulin and NPH injected in the morning, with regular or rapid-acting insulin injected before dinner and NPH at bedtime. It is designed to reduce the risk for nocturnal hypoglycemia and counteract the dawn phenomenon (**Figure 8.10**). However, the patient may need a small amount of NPH administered at dinnertime to provide sufficient basal insulin between the waning of the rapid-acting dinnertime insulin and the bedtime injection of NPH.

Establishing the Correct Insulin Dose

Achieving stringent glycemic control entails determining the total daily dose (TDD) of insulin. Once this foundation is established, basal, prandial, and correction doses can be closely estimated, and more refined dose adjustments can be made by analyzing glucose patterns.

Following is a general formula for establishing an initial regimen in the newly diagnosed patient with type 1 diabetes (**Table 8.3**). It is intended only as a general guideline and must be adapted to the patient's indi-

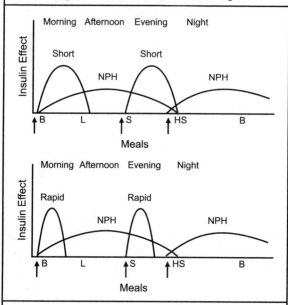

FIGURE 8.10 — Schematic Representation of Idealized Insulin Effect Provided by a Regimen of Alternating Intermediate-Acting With Short- or Rapid-Acting Insulins in Morning, Predinner, and Bedtime Injections

Abbreviations: B, breakfast; HS, bedtime; L, lunch; NPH, neutral protamine Hagedorn [insulin]; S, supper.

Schematic representation of idealized insulin effect provided by a regimen consisting of a morning injection of intermediate-acting insulin (NPH) and short- (*top*) or rapid (*bottom*) acting insulin, a predinner injection of short- (*top*) or rapid- (*bottom*) acting insulin, and a bedtime injection of intermediate-acting insulin. Arrows indicate time of insulin injection.

Klingensmith G, ed, for the American Diabetes Association. *Intensive Diabetes Management.* 3rd ed. New York, NY: The McGraw-Hill Companies; 2003:90.

TABLE 8.3 — Establishing Initial Insulin Regimen in Newly Diagnosed Patients With Type 1 Diabetes

Calculate Total Daily Dose (TDD)
TDD = 0.3 U (average for full insulin replacement in type 1 patients, 0.7; range, 0.3 to 1.0 U) × body weight (kg)

Calculate Basal Insulin Requirement
Basal insulin requirement = 40% to 50% of TDD

The dose may be advanced every 2 to 3 days for NPH and weekly for Ultralente and insulin glargine.

Calculate Mealtime Insulin Doses
Total mealtime insulin dose = TDD – basal insulin requirement

The prebreakfast, prelunch, and predinner doses will depend on the number of calories consumed at each meal and the type of insulin used.

Calculate Correction Dose
If the patient's insulin sensitivity is unknown, it is wise to start with a conservative dose, eg, 1 U/50 mg/dL, and titrate upward based on the results of blood glucose testing. On average, 1 U of short-acting insulin lowers blood glucose about 30 mg/dL (range, 20 mg/dL to 70 mg/dL).

Adapted from: Zinman B. *Clin Cornerstone*. 1998;3:29-38.

vidual needs. Note that initial doses are intentionally conservative and almost always have to be increased:

- Calculate the patient's TDD of insulin, ie, the sum of all units of all types of insulin taken. To determine the TDD in a newly diagnosed patient, multiply the patient's body weight in kilograms by 0.3 U (average for full insulin replacement in patients with type 1 diabetes, 0.7 U/kg, range, 0.3 U/kg to 1.0 U/kg). For example, if the patient weighs 100 kg, the TDD = 30 U.

- Determine the basal insulin requirement. This should be 40% to 50% of the TDD. The basal insulin requirement may be in the form of NPH, Lente, Ultralente, or insulin glargine. The dose may be advanced every 2 to 3 days for NPH and weekly for Ultralente and insulin glargine.
- Determine the prandial insulin requirement. The total prandial insulin dose is equal to the TDD minus the basal insulin dose. For example, if the TDD were 30 U and the basal insulin requirement were 12 U (30 × 0.4), the total mealtime dose would be 18 U. The prebreakfast, prelunch, and predinner doses will depend on the number of calories consumed at each meal and the type of insulin used.
- Determine the correction dose. If the patient's insulin sensitivity is unknown, it is wise to start with a conservative dose (eg, 1 U/50 mg/dL) and titrate upward based on the results of blood glucose testing. On average, 1 U of short-acting insulin will lower blood glucose approximately 30 to 50 mg/dL (range 20 to 70 mg/dL).

■ **Special Situations**

Newly diagnosed patients with type 1 diabetes may experience some pancreatic β-cell function within a few weeks of diagnosis. This is known as "the honeymoon period," during which episodes of hypoglycemia could ensue if the insulin dose is not decreased (eg, 0.2 to 0.6 U/kg/day). Blood glucose levels should be monitored frequently during this period, and patients should take the highest dose of insulin that does not cause hypoglycemia.

Insulin needs may be higher than usual in patients who are ill and also during pregnancy when doses should be progressively increased (in units per kilogram) to accommodate weight gain. The adolescent growth spurt is another period of elevated insulin requirements (1.3 to 1.5 U/kg/day), and this greater need could continue throughout puberty.

Adjusting Insulin Regimens

Insulin adjustments are made when individualized blood glucose targets are not being met. Any plan of action should be based on SMBG determinations and daily records. Actions may involve altering the timing of insulin injections, changing the dosage, or revising the content of meals. Among these alternatives, most patients find adjusting insulin dosages most convenient. If blood glucose levels are exceptionally low, however, adjusting carbohydrate intake may be warranted; and for unusually high levels, postponing mealtime after insulin administration may be necessary.

Correction doses of insulin are used for acute adjustments in response to immediate circumstances. The correction dose is added to the usual prandial and basal doses. Nevertheless, recurring problems of blood glucose levels outside the target range should be addressed by a change in treatment regimen rather than by continual supplemental insulin doses. Such changes are referred to as pattern adjustments.

■ Determining the Correction Dose

The need for a correction dose of insulin may be assessed on the basis of the following criteria:
- Current blood glucose level
- Intended amount of carbohydrate consumption
- Degree of activity planned after eating
- Degree of activity within the hour prior to eating
- History of changes in blood glucose under similar circumstances.

The typical intervention is an adjustment in the insulin dose, although alterations in activity, food intake, and timing of insulin administration may also be appropriate (see *Establishing the Correct Insulin Dose* in preceding section). Examples of these adjustments are shown in **Table 8.4**. The patient's individual correction factor (ie, the extent to which blood glucose will decrease per unit of rapid-acting insulin based on premeal blood glucose levels) must be determined to adjust prandial insulin doses properly. Although there is no exact method for calculating the correction factor (also referred to as the "insulin sensitivity" factor), many clinicians employ the "1800 Rule" if using rapid-acting insulin (or the "1500 Rule" for regular insulin) (**Table 8.5**). The correction factor may also be applied to between-meal elevations in blood glucose.

Patients using lispro, aspart, or glulisine should periodically test the accuracy of their correction factor by taking the following steps:

- Select a premeal target, usually between 90 and 140 mg/dL
- Begin the test when blood glucose is >200 mg/dL, provided it has been at least 4 to 5 hours since the last dose of insulin was given (or 6 to 8 hours if regular insulin is being used), and at least 2 hours since food was eaten
- Determine how many milligrams per deciliter to drop by subtracting the target blood glucose from the current blood glucose
- Divide the desired drop in milligrams per deciliter by the correction factor to determine the correction dose (eg, if the blood glucose 5 hours after the last dose of lispro is 240 mg/dL and the target is 120 mg/dL, the correction factor should be 1 U/40 mg/dL, and, hence, the correction dose = (240 to 120 mg/dL)/40 mg/dL = 3 U of insulin lispro)
- Inject the correction dose and monitor blood glucose every hour (or more often) to catch and treat possible hypoglycemia

TABLE 8.4 — Sample Plan for Premeal Dosing of Rapid-Acting Insulin Analogue (Lispro/Aspart/Glulisine)*

Using an insulin-to-carbohydrate ratio for meal insulin dose if blood glucose is:
- <50/dL
  - Reduce premeal insulin analogue by 2 to 3 U, or
  - Delay injection until 10 to 15 minutes after starting to eat, or
  - Include at least 15 g of rapidly available carbohydrate at the start of the meal
- 70 to 130 mg/dL
  - Take prescribed premeal dose of insulin analogue
- 250 to 300 mg/dL
  - Increase premeal insulin analogue by 4 U, or
  - Consider delaying meal to 10 to 20 minutes after injection

For a constant carbohydrate diet with a fixed-insulin dose for the meal:
- If the planned meal is larger than usual, increase insulin analogue by 1 to 2 U
- If the planned meal is smaller than usual, decrease insulin analogue by 1 to 2 U

Adjustment for exercise:
- If unusually increased activity is planned after eating, eat extra carbohydrate and/or decrease insulin analogue by 10% to 20%
- If unusually sedentary activity is planned after eating, consider increasing insulin analogue by 10% to 20%

* This plan assumes that the preprandial and bedtime blood glucose target is 70 to 30 mg/dL (3.9-7.2 mmol/L) or a mean target of 100 mg/dL (5.6 mmol/L) and the correction dose is 1 U/50 mg/dL. Plans should be individualized for each patient. Once the insulin dosage is stable, use the following scheme for premeal alteration of the insulin dose.

Klingensmith GJ, ed, for the American Diabetes Association. *Intensive Diabetes Management*. 3rd ed. Alexandria, Va: American Diabetes Association; 2003.

TABLE 8.5 — The "1800/1500 Rules"		
Total Daily Insulin Dose (U)	**1800 Rule:** Drop in BG per Unit of Lispro/Aspart/ Glulisine (mg/dL)	**1500 Rule:** Drop in BG per Unit of Regular (mg/dL)
20	90	75
25	72	60
30	60	50
35	51	43
40	45	38
50	36	30
60	30	25
75	24	20
100	18	15
Abbreviation: BG, blood glucose.		
Adapted from: Walsh J, Roberts R, eds. *Insulin Pump Therapy Handbook*. Sylmar, Calif: MiniMed, Inc; 1992:34.		

- If after 6 hours of fasting, the blood glucose level is within 30 mg/dL of the target, the correction factor can be considered accurate.

If the correction factor differs significantly from the amount predicted, the TDD or basal insulin dose may be incorrect.

■ Pattern Adjustments

When blood glucose levels are consistently above or below target range at a particular time of the day, it may be necessary to make prospective changes in the insulin regimen based on analysis of past blood glucose patterns. SMBG records should be evaluated every 3 to 7 days to discern the timing of recurrent episodes of hyperglycemia or hypoglycemia. The prandial component of the insulin regimen should be analyzed first, followed by the basal component. **Table**

8.6 shows examples of changes that may be made to correct frequent highs and lows in blood glucose levels. For a more detailed discussion of pattern management, see Chapter 11, *Using Blood Glucose Data Technology for Pattern Management.*

■ Adjusting for Diet and Exercise
Diet

Adjusting prandial insulin doses for variations in food intake is fundamental to stringent glycemic control. The commonly used formula calls for 1 U of insulin per 10 to 15 g of carbohydrate. In practice, however, the ratio can range from 0.5 to 2.0 U for every 10 to 15 g of carbohydrate. In general, the more carbohydrate in a meal, the larger the dose needed; and a higher TDD will necessitate a larger dose to cover a specific amount of carbohydrate.

Matching insulin to carbohydrate intake is easier with the insulin analogues lispro, aspart, and glulisine than with regular insulin, which has a slower onset of action and longer duration of effect. To estimate how many grams of carbohydrate are covered by 1 U of lispro, aspart, or glulisine a value referred to as the carbohydrate factor, it is useful to use the "500 Rule":

$$500 \div \text{TDD} = \text{grams of carbohydrate covered by 1 U insulin}$$

For example, a person who uses 50 U of insulin per day will need 1 U for every 10 g of carbohydrate (500 $\div$ 50 U = 10). If that person consumes two slices of bread containing 15 g each, it will take 3 U of lispro, aspart, or glulisine to cover these 30 g of carbohydrates. This rule is most accurate for patients with type 1 diabetes who receive 50% to 60% of their TDD as basal insulin and who are replacing basal and prandial insulin separately after having accurately determined their TDD. For those who are not using a basal/

TABLE 8.6 — Sample Adjustments in Insulin Regimen Based on Results of Self-Monitoring of Blood Glucose

Hyperglycemia
- Fasting
  - Increase evening intermediate-acting or long-acting insulin
  - Decrease evening snack
- Prelunch
  - Increase morning dose of short-acting insulin
  - Decrease size or carbohydrate component of breakfast
  - Increase activity level in morning
- Predinner
  - Increase dose of morning intermediate-acting or pre-lunch short-acting insulin
  - Decrease size or carbohydrate component of lunch
  - Increase activity level in afternoon
- Bedtime
  - Increase dose of evening short-acting insulin
  - Decrease size or carbohydrate component of dinner
  - Increase activity level after dinner

Hypoglycemia
- Fasting
  - Decrease evening intermediate-acting or long-acting insulin
- Prelunch
  - Decrease morning dose of short-acting insulin
  - Increase size or carbohydrate component of breakfast
- Predinner
  - Decrease morning dose of intermediate-acting or pre-lunch short-acting insulin
  - Increase size or carbohydrate component of lunch
- Bedtime
  - Decrease evening short-acting insulin dose
  - Increase size or carbohydrate component of dinner

Adapted from: American Diabetes Association. *Medical Management of Type 1 Diabetes*. Alexandria, Va: American Diabetes Association; 1998.

prandial approach, ie, are on two injections per day with the morning basal insulin covering lunchtime carbohydrate consumption, the 500 Rule can be used only as a rough guideline.

Another way to determine the carbohydrate factor is to add all the carbohydrates eaten and divide this number by the total units of prandial insulin used per day for 3 days. For example, if 300 g of carbohydrate are consumed per day and 30 U of lispro are needed to cover them, the carb factor would be calculated as: $300 \div 10 = 10$ g per unit or 1 U for every 10 g of carbohydrate. This method can be simpler and works well for patients who have a fixed routine of meals and snacks each day.

Prandial insulin to cover carbohydrate intake may be reduced or skipped entirely when:

- Extra carbohydrates are eaten to raise low blood glucose levels
- Extra carbohydrates are eaten to cover increased physical activity
- Nausea or vomiting may prevent the patient from keeping carbohydrates down.

NOTE: Even if prandial insulin is decreased or eliminated, basal and correction dose insulins must be continued.

When determining prandial insulin adjustments, it is necessary to consider the time of the last insulin injection. If using regular insulin and the last injection was <8 hours prior, some percentage of activity from that insulin will still be in effect; therefore, the supplemental insulin dose may have to be established with that in mind. This is less of a problem with rapid-acting insulin because peak activity is reached within 2 hours. In general, some activity from the rapid-acting analogues will still be available for 4 to 5 hours after the last injection.

Exercise

For light exercise that lasts under an hour, eating extra carbohydrates is the most straightforward approach to keeping blood glucose levels within target range. However, lowering the insulin level will enable fuel to be released from glycogen and fat stores in lieu of eating extra carbohydrates for fuel. This approach helps patients who want to lose weight or participate in long periods of intense physical activity without consuming large portions of carbohydrates.

As exercise becomes longer and more vigorous, a reduction in insulin dose will be necessary. Whether prandial or basal doses should be reduced depends on the duration of the activity, its timing in relation to meals, and whether the exercise was planned. Any reduction in insulin doses must take into account the lag time before insulin in the blood actually begins to wane.

A reduction in prandial doses of lispro, aspart, or glulisine is warranted when exercise is moderate or strenuous, lasts <90 minutes, and begins within 90 minutes of a meal. When strenuous exercise lasts >60 minutes or moderate exercise 90 minutes, a reduction in the basal dose should be considered as well. Basal reductions typically should be initiated several hours before exercise begins. **Table 8.7** shows how long before exercise each type of insulin should be reduced.

The aforementioned 500 Rule may be used to reduce insulin doses by following these steps:
- Divide the TDD into 500 to determine the patient's carbohydrate factor.
- Determine how many carbohydrates will be needed for the planned exercise, as shown in **Table 8.8**.
- Divide the carbohydrates required for exercise by the carbohydrate factor to calculate the ratio of insulin to exercise.

TABLE 8.7 — Timing of Insulin Dose Reduction Before Exercise

Type of Insulin	Length of Time Before Exercise to Begin Dosage Reduction	Duration of Effect (hours)
Lispro/aspart/ glulisine	15 to 20 minutes	3.5
Regular	30 to 45 minutes	5
NPH or Lente	2 to 4 hours	14
Ultralente	3 to 4 hours	18
Insulin glargine	2 to 4 hours	20

Adapted from: Walsh J, et al. *Using Insulin: Everything You Need for Success With Insulin.* San Diego, Calif: Torrey Pines Press; 2003:243.

- Having determined both the carbohydrate and insulin equivalents of the planned exercise, the patient may choose to eat extra carbohydrates, lower the prandial insulin dose, or both.

It is necessary to keep in mind that insulin doses must be reduced with caution and always under the advice of the health care team. Blood glucose levels should be tested often during and after exercise, and fast carbohydrates, like glucose tablets, should be carried at all times for rapid correction of low blood glucose.

Injection Devices

Concern about injections is often a deterrent to initiating multiple-component insulin regimens aimed at meticulous glycemic control. However, currently available injection devices eliminate or reduce many of the problems formerly associated with SC administration of insulin. Insulin pens are especially useful in multicomponent regimens because they are convenient to carry and eliminate the need to draw up insulin frequently throughout the day. They are particularly well-suited to extremely insulin-sensitive patients, such as children and thin adult women. The penlike device holds insulin cartridges containing 300 U of regular, lispro, aspart, NPH, 75/25, or 70/30. Disposable needles are attached to the end of the insulin pen. The desired dose is administered by turning a dial selector, injecting the needle, and pushing a button at the end of the pen to inject the insulin.

Spring-loaded designs hold conventional insulin syringes. When activated by the patient, the device injects the needle. However, this form of delivery may result in variable insulin action due to inconsistent penetration of the insulin into the fat and muscle tissue. Another innovation is the use of small needles or catheters with an external injection port that can be implanted into the abdomen and left there for several days. Injections are then given through the catheter instead of the skin, thereby minimizing needle punctures.

SUGGESTED READING

Bolli GB. Physiological insulin replacement in type 1 diabetes mellitus. *Exp Clin Endocrinol Diabetes.* 2001;109 (suppl 2):S317-S332.

Burge MR, Schade DS. Insulins. *Endocrinol Metab Clin North Am.* 1997;26:575-598.

DeWitt DE, Hirsch IB. Outpatient insulin therapy in type 1 and type 2 diabetes mellitus: scientific review. *JAMA.* 2003;289:2254-2264.

Heise T, Heinemann L. Rapid and long-acting analogues as an approach to improve insulin therapy: an evidence-based medicine assessment. *Curr Pharm Des.* 2001;7:1303-1325.

Hirsch IB. Type 1 diabetes mellitus and the use of flexible insulin regimens. *Am Fam Physician.* 1999;60:2343-2356.

TABLE 8.8 — Grams of Carbohydrate Used per Hour for Various Activities

Activity	Patient Weight			% Calories From Carbohydrates
	100 lb	150 lb	200 lb	
Baseball	25	38	50	40
Running				
5 mph	45	68	90	50
8 mph	96	145	190	65
10 mph	126	189	252	70
Bicycling				
6 mph	20	27	34	40
10 mph	35	48	61	50
14 mph	60	83	105	60
18 mph	95	130	165	65
20 mph	122	168	214	70

Walking				
3 mph	15	22	29	30
4.5 mph	30	45	59	45
Mopping	16	23	30	30
Raking leaves	19	28	38	30
Swimming				
Slow crawl	41	56	71	50
Fast crawl	69	95	121	60

Adapted from: Walsh J, et al. *Using Insulin: Everything You Need for Success With Insulin.* San Diego, Calif: Torrey Pines Press; 2003:239.

Home PD, Lindholm A, Riis A, European Insulinn Aspart Study Group. Insulin aspart vs human insulin in the management of long-term blood glucose control in type 1 diabetes mellitus: a randomized controlled trial. *Diabet Med.* 2000;17:762-770.

Klingensmith GJ, ed. *Intensive Diabetes Management.* 3rd ed. Alexandria, Va: American Diabetes Association; 2003.

Lalli C, Ciofetta M, Del Sindaco P, et al. Long-term intensive treatment of type 1 diabetes with the short-acting insulin analog lispro in variable combination with NPH insulin at mealtime. *Diabetes Care.* 1999;22:468-477.

Owens DR, Zinman B, Bolli GB. Insulins today and beyond. *Lancet.* 2001;358:739-746.

Ratner RE, Hirsch IB, Neifing JL, Garg SK, Mecca TE, Wilson CA. Less hypoglycemia with insulin glargine in intensive insulin therapy for type 1 diabetes. US Study Group of Insulin Glargine in Type 1 Diabetes. *Diabetes Care.* 2000;23:639-643.

Rosenstock J, Park G, Zimmerman J, U.S. Insulin Glargine (HOE 901) Type 1 Diabetes Investigator Group. Basal insulin glargine (HOE 901) versus NPH insulin in patients with type 1 diabetes on multiple daily insulin regimens. *Diabetes Care.* 2000;23:1127-1142.

Rossetti P, Pampanelli S, Fanelli C, et al. Intensive replacement of basal insulin in patients with type 1 diabetes given rapid-acting insulin analog at mealtime: a 3-month comparison between administration of NPH insulin four times daily and glargine insulin at dinner or bedtime. *Diabetes Care.* 2003;26:1490-1496.

Walsh J, Roberts R, Bailey T, Varma CB. *Using Insulin: Everything You Need for Success With Insulin.* San Diego, Calif: Torrey Pines Press; 2003.

White JR Jr, Campbell RK, Hirsch IB. Novel insulins and strict glycemic control. Analogues approximate normal insulin secretory response. *Postgrad Med.* 2003;113:30-36.

9 Continuous Subcutaneous Insulin Infusion

Continuous subcutaneous insulin infusion (CSII), often referred to as insulin pump therapy, was developed in the late 1970s as a research tool to improve glycemic control in difficult-to-control patients with type 1 diabetes. Although the technology has changed over the years and models have varied, the basic device uses a portable electromechanical pump that attempts to replicate physiologic insulin delivery. Fast-acting insulin analogues are infused into the subcutaneous (SC) tissue at preprogrammed rates over 24 hours, and patient-determined boluses are given before meals. In the 1980s, initial enthusiasm for CSII as an alternative to insulin injections eventually gave way to concerns about the size, safety, cost, and efficacy of pump therapy. There was a resurgence of interest during the 1990s when publication of the Diabetes Control and Complications Trial (DCCT) showed that near-normalization of glycemia with intensive therapy could prevent the development and slow the progression of diabetes-related complications. In addition, Nicole Johnson, who was Miss America in 1999, wore an insulin pump during the pageant and helped to bolster popularity. Use of pumps has continued to grow, with >200,000 people using pumps in the United States.

For both clinical and economic reasons, efforts have been under way to clearly delineate the advantages and disadvantages of CSII and to determine which patients stand to gain the most from this relatively more expensive treatment choice. It is hoped that by establishing clear clinical guidelines for CSII (based on audits of factors such as the clinical reasons for starting pump therapy, its metabolic effectiveness, possible side effects, impact on long-term complications, quality of life, and choice of treatment modalities), specific patient populations will have greater access to this therapeutic option.

Benefits of CSII

CSII offers several important clinical and quality-of-life benefits compared with other forms of insulin delivery (**Table 9**.**1**). Patients who opt for CSII are usually seeking a more flexible lifestyle that simultaneously affords better glycemic control. CSII is the most precise way to mimic normal insulin secretion because basal rates can be programmed in half-hour segments throughout a 24-hour period and boluses given on demand with meals based on carbohydrate counting, correction factors, and prior experience (**Figure 9**.**1**). Essentially, the CSII pump may be thought of as a computerized mechanical syringe automatically delivering insulin in physiologic fashion. Patients can

---

TABLE 9.1 — Benefits of Continuous Subcutaneous Insulin Infusion

Clinical Benefits
- Improved glycemic control
- Control of the dawn phenomenon
- Fewer glycemic excursions
- Improved growth and development in poorly controlled adolescents with type 1 diabetes

Quality-of-Life Benefits
- Flexibility in meal timing and amounts
- Fewer and less severe hypoglycemic reactions
- Increased flexibility in exercise intensity and times
- Improved control while traveling
- Improved control with variable work schedule
- Greater self-reliance

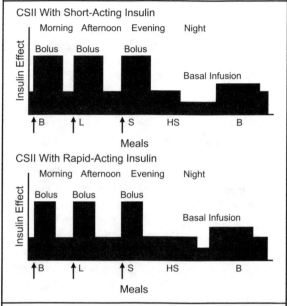

FIGURE 9.1 — Schematic Representation of Idealized Insulin Effect Provided by Continuous Subcutaneous Insulin Infusion Therapy With Short- or Rapid-Acting Insulin

Abbreviations: B, breakfast; HS, bedtime; L, lunch; S, supper.

Schematic representation of idealized insulin effect provided by CSII of short- (*top*) or rapid- (*bottom*) acting insulin. Arrows indicate time of premeal insulin bolus.

Klingensmith GJ, ed, for the American Diabetes Association. *Intensive Diabetes Management*. 3rd ed. New York, NY: The McGraw-Hill Companies; 2003:87.

accommodate metabolic changes related to eating, exercise, illness, or varying work and travel schedules by modifying insulin availability on a minute-to-minute basis. Basal rates can also be adjusted to match lower insulin demands at night and higher ones to accommodate for the dawn phenomenon requirements between approximately 3 AM or 4 AM and 8 AM. Further-more, because pumps use only rapid-acting and short-acting insulin, the vagaries of insulin absorption and pharmacokinetics, which are responsible for up to 50% to 60% of the day-to-day fluctuation in blood glucose, are improved.

Various studies comparing glycemic control during CSII vs intensive insulin injection regimens have been published. A meta-analysis of 12 randomized controlled trials of CSII vs multiple-injection regimens showed a weighted mean difference in blood glucose concentration of 16.2 mg/dL (95% confidence interval [CI], 0.5–1.2) and a difference in A1C of 0.5% (0.2–0.7) favoring CSII. The slightly but significantly better control in patients on CSII was accomplished with a 14% average reduction in daily insulin dose.

A large body of evidence suggests that hypoglycemia is significantly less common with CSII than with multiple-injection therapy, even when the injection regimen is not intensive. In a study of 40 type 1 diabetic patients, the frequency of hypoglycemic coma during CSII was less than one third that in a comparable group of patients treated with insulin injections. Similarly, in a randomized crossover trial of CSII vs insulin injection therapy, the number of mild and moderate hypoglycemic episodes (severe hypoglycemia did not occur) was reduced nearly 60% by CSII. Moreover, retrospective analysis of medical records at an academic diabetes clinic revealed not only a marked reduction in the frequency of severe hypoglycemic episodes among 107 patients with type 1 diabetes using CSII, but also significantly improved glycemic control (**Figure 9.2** and **Figure 9.3**).

Mechanics of CSII

Modern insulin pumps are much smaller and easier to use than the pumps of a decade ago. Most

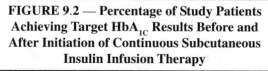

FIGURE 9.2 — Percentage of Study Patients Achieving Target HbA$_{1C}$ Results Before and After Initiation of Continuous Subcutaneous Insulin Infusion Therapy

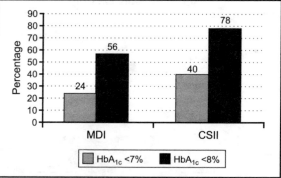

Abbreviations: CSII, continuous subcutaneous insulin infusion; HbA$_{1C}$, glycosylated hemoglobin; MDI, multiple daily injections.

Rudoph JW, Hirsch IB. *Endocr Pract.* 2002;8:404.

weigh around 115 g (4 oz) and are approximately the size of a small cellular phone or pager. Each houses an insulin-filled cartridge or syringe connected to a 23- to 24-inch, 31-inch, or 42- to 43-inch length of plastic tubing (**Figure 9.4**). At the end of the tubing is a 25- or 27-gauge needle or a soft Teflon cannula that can be inserted into the SC tissue at a 30- to 45- or 90-degree angle, depending on the type of infusion set used. The abdomen is the preferred infusion site because placement of the needle there is convenient and comfortable and insulin absorption is most consistent in that region. However, the upper outer quadrant of the buttocks, upper thighs, and triceps fat pad of the arms may also be used.

Most infusion sets now allow removal of the needle, leaving only the soft flexible cannula in place subcutaneously, whereas the older infusion sets require

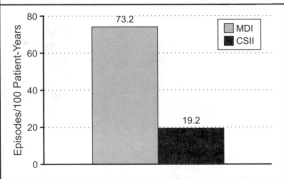

FIGURE 9.3 — Comparison of Severe Hypoglycemic Episodes in Study Patients During Multiple Daily Injections of Insulin and Continuous Subcutaneous Insulin Infusion Therapy

Abbreviations: CSII, continuous subcutaneous insulin infusion; MDI, multiple daily injections.

Percentage change in hypoglycemic events was -73.8% ($P = 0.0003$).

Rudoph JW, Hirsch IB. *Endocr Pract.* 2002;8:404.

that the needle remain under the skin. After the syringe is placed in the pump, a lever mechanically pushes down the plunger of the syringe, and the insulin travels through the infusion tube, entering the SC tissue through either the implanted bent needle or the soft, flexible catheter. In current models, infusion lines have a quick-release mechanism, allowing them to be temporarily disconnected from the insertion site. This quick-release feature makes dressing, swimming, showering, and other activities more convenient.

Only regular or fast-acting insulin should be used in insulin pumps. The basal rate of the insulin pump replaces the intermediate- and longer-acting insulins, such as NPH, Ultralente, and glargine. The boluses of aspart and lispro are given before each meal and are

FIGURE 9.4 — Insulin Infusion Pumps and Subcutaneous Catheter Infusion Sets

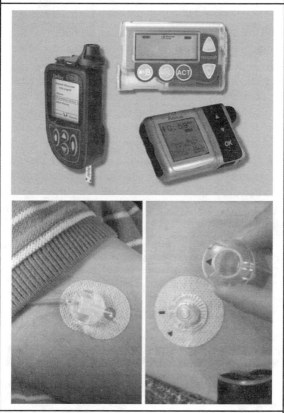

Examples of three insulin infusion pumps *(top)* and two available infusion lines that feature quick release functioning to allow for various activities, such as taking a shower *(bottom)*.

essentially determined the same way as with a multiple-injection regimen. The pump allows programming of many different basal infusion rates (usually ranging from 0.4 to 2.0 U/hour) to meet nonprandial basal insulin requirements. The average patient will require no more than one to two different basal rates throughout the day or night. In addition to covering meals and snacks, the bolus mode can be used to correct incidental hyperglycemia resulting from increased food intake, illness, or stress. Unfortunately, current insulin pumps do not have glucose sensors to automatically signal the pump when more or less insulin is needed, but this technology may be available within the next few years as sensor technology matures. Built-in alarms alert the patient in the event that insulin delivery occurs inadvertently or is disrupted for any reason. **Table 9**.2 lists some important features to consider when selecting an insulin pump. Pump manufacturer representatives and manufacturers' web sites are good sources of information when comparing the different models. Manufacturers of insulin pumps in the United States are:

- Animas Corporation (www.animascorp.com)
- DANA Diabecare USA (www.danapumps.com)
- Smiths Medical MD, Inc (formerly Deltec, Inc) (www.cozmore.com)
- Medtronic MiniMed (www.minimed.com)
- Nipro Diabetes Systems (www.nipro-diabetes.com).

Initiating CSII Therapy

Ideally, CSII should be initiated with the help of an educated and motivated health care team, including a diabetes educator proficient in pump therapy. However, because of third-party reimbursement, outpatient initiation provides a good opportunity for integrating pump therapy into the patient's daily routine and is more practical than inpatient initiation. Before beginning therapy, it will be necessary to review the topics listed in **Table 9.3** with the patient. Frequent contact for the first 2 to 3 days is necessary to ensure that the patient is comfortable with the mechanics of the pump, that bolus and basal rates are set appropri-

TABLE 9.2 — Selected Therapeutic and Safety Features of Pumps (Depending on Model)

- The basal rate can be adjusted temporarily for periods of increased activity, illness, or stress without changing the usual basal rate program
- Basal delivery can be suspended if necessary; an "auto-off" feature suspends insulin delivery if no programming occurs within a set period of time
- Several basal rate patterns (2 to 4, depending on the pump model) can be programmed for easy switching between patterns
- Boluses and their time of delivery can be reviewed
- Boluses can be programmed via voice
- Total daily insulin delivery and alarm history can be monitored
- An extended or square-wave bolus feature that allows delivery of a bolus over a prolonged period (ranging from 15 minutes to 8 hours, depending on the model)
- Alarm system for low/dead battery, empty cartridge/syringe, occlusion, pump delivery error, and electronic malfunction; tamper-resistant blocks
- Backlight display
- Watertight or water-resistant
- Remote programmer
- Software to integrate history data with data stored in blood glucose meters, plus data summaries and graphs
- Programmability to and from a personal computer

Adapted from: American Diabetes Association. *Intensive Diabetes Management*. 3rd ed. Alexandria, Va: American Diabetes Association; 2003:103.

ately, and that the patient is monitoring blood glucose frequently and at appropriate times. Blood glucose should be measured before and 1 to 2 hours after each meal, at bedtime, and at 3 AM to help determine preprandial rates as well as continuous basal rates during a typical 24-hour period.

The initial bolus and basal rates can be set according to the patient's prior insulin regimen. If the patient

> ### TABLE 9.3 — Topics to Review With Patients Before Initiating Continuous Subcutaneous Insulin Infusion
>
> - Target goals for glucose control
> - Prevention of diabetic ketoacidosis
> - Prevention of hypoglycemia
> - Insulin pump and infusion set operation (catheter care)
> - Guidelines for basal rate and bolus adjustment
> - Sick-day rules
> - Troubleshooting for unexplained hyperglycemia

has had reasonably good glycemic control, the prepump total daily dose (TDD) should be reduced by 10% to 25% before calculating a starting basal rate because insulin requirements often decrease with pump therapy. Alternatively, the basal rate may be calculated by dividing 50% of the total combined insulin requirements by 24 hours, again keeping in mind that this rate will need to be reduced 10% to 25% once the patient is using the pump. For example, a patient whose total daily combined insulin dose is 50 U would calculate the basal insulin dose as 25 U divided by 24 hours equaling approximately 1.0 U/hour; and with a 20% reduction, the initial basal rate would be 0.8 U/hour.

Calculation of the basal rate can also be estimated or confirmed by multiplying the patient's weight in kilograms by 0.22 U. For example, if a patient weighs 80 kg, the basal rate should be 0.7 U/hour (80 kg × 0.22 U ÷ 24 hours). If the results are not consistent, the lowest rate should be chosen initially. In general, patients with type 1 diabetes require basal rates within the range of 0.4 to 2.0 U/hour, with the average adult requiring 0.5 to 1.0 U/kg body weight/day. The timing for the discontinuation of the patient's intermediate-acting or long-acting insulin needs to be managed properly so that there is little overlap of both therapies and to avoid insulinopenia as well. For example, if a patient is on 20 U of insulin glargine (Lantus) at bedtime, the insulin pump should be initiated approximately 20 to 24 hours after the last injection. Frequent glucose monitoring is required to make adjustments if needed.

Verifying the Basal Rate

To verify the overnight basal rate, the patient should avoid eating food after dinner and test the level of blood glucose 2 hours after dinner, at bedtime, at 3 AM, and first thing in the morning. If these values are higher or lower than desired, adjust the basal rate accordingly, usually by increments of 0.05 to 0.20 U/hour. If the 3 AM and fasting blood glucose levels are widely different, the basal rates during sleep and early morning (before waking) may require adjustment. Certain situations may give clinical clues to be used for adjusting the daytime rate. For example, if the patient becomes hypoglycemic when meals are skipped or delayed, the daytime basal rate may be too high; or, if the 2-hour postprandial blood glucose value is within target range, but the premeal reading is not, the basal rate may be too low. A patient can also have an early breakfast and fast all day until a late dinner to determine if the basal rate is adequate during the day.

Determining Prandial (Bolus) Rates

Anyone undertaking CSII should know how to calculate their preprandial insulin dose according to the grams of carbohydrate consumed at each meal or snack. This means that patients should be able to match the meal boluses to the intake of carbohydrate with an individualized ratio of 1 U of insulin per some specified amount of carbohydrate, referred to as the insulin-to-carbohydrate ratio. The method for determining the insulin-to-carbohydrate ratio is explained in Chapter 8, *Multiple-Component Insulin Therapy*. A suggested starting ratio is 1 U of insulin for every 10 to 15 g carbohydrate for adults and 1 U insulin for every 20 to 30 g carbohydrate for children or insulin-sensitive adults.

As with all intensive insulin regimens, conscientious blood glucose monitoring is essential to determine the effectiveness of insulin dosages relative to carbohydrate counting and the patient's level of physical activity. Blood glucose testing should be performed initially before eating, within 1 to 2 hours following the start of each meal, at bedtime, and at 3 AM until glycemic goals are achieved. Additional adjustments may be needed in response to specific circumstances. At minimum, blood glucose testing should be done four times per day (before meals and at bedtime) and once weekly around 3 AM.

If an adjustment of rapid-acting or regular insulin is needed to correct premeal or between-meal hyperglycemia, patients can use the "1800 Rule" (the "1500 Rule" in the case of regular insulin) to calculate their insulin sensitivity factor (or correction factor), as described in the preceding chapter. This can be done by dividing 1800 or 1500, depending on the type of insulin used, by the TDD of insulin. For example, a patient using insulin lispro whose TDD is 50 U has an insulin sensitivity factor of 36 mg/dL ($1800 \div 50 = 36$ mg/dL). Thus 1 U of rapid-acting insulin decreases this patient's blood glucose by 36 mg/dL. Additionally, if the patient is using regular insulin and the premeal blood glucose level is elevated, administering the bolus 45 to 60 minutes before the meal can further improve glycemic control. (For more information on insulin adjustments in response to diet, exercise, and illness, refer to Chapter 7, *Nonpharmacologic Management*.) It is important to emphasize that the formulas merely give us best estimates of what the patient will require; only with trial and error will the

126

patient be able to fine tune the insulin-to-carbohydrate ratio and correction factor.

After initiation of CSII, the patient should be contacted daily for the first 3 or 4 days to discuss blood glucose values and address any questions. Once bolus and basal rates are sufficiently adjusted to achieve glycemic goals, the patient can be seen in 2 to 4 weeks. The diabetes educators contracted by the different pump companies are usually excellent at keeping in close touch with the patient and reporting important information back to the caregiver.

Risks of CSII

■ Unexplained Hyperglycemia and Ketoacidosis

Patients new to CSII must be taught to suspect interrupted insulin delivery any time high blood glucose levels persist in the absence of illness or any other circumstance that might affect glycemia. Often the first sign is an inexplicably elevated blood glucose reading during a routine check. If the blood glucose level remains above target 2 to 4 hours later, especially if additional insulin has been administered, disruption of insulin delivery is the likely cause and measures should be taken to avoid ketoacidosis, a potentially life-threatening condition that occurs in the absence of adequate insulin (see Chapter 13, *Acute Complications*).

If the cause of the problem cannot be explained by an alteration in the treatment regimen, the patient should examine the pump/syringe/infusion set system and site for any obvious source of malfunction. If there is a problem with the site, the infusion set or tubing, or the connection between the syringe and the infusion site, the catheter and site should be changed. If a problem with the pump is detected, the pump should be reprogrammed or replaced. If there is partial or complete occlusion of insulin in the infusion set or site, replacing the cartridge/syringe and infusion set or

127

changing the site may help. Sometimes simply using a new vial of insulin will correct the problem because insulin can lose potency over time. On the back of all insulin pumps, there is a toll-free 24-hour hotline phone number for questions and/or problems.

If the problem is not easily resolved, patients should use a multiple-injection regimen until the pump can be replaced. Extra insulin, pump supplies, and conventional syringes or insulin pens should be accessible at all times, and patients should know how to switch to an injection regimen if necessary. Intermediate-acting or long-acting insulin should be available for these infrequent episodes. Additionally, patients should monitor blood glucose and urine ketone levels every 1 to 3 hours and administer insulin boluses via injection until urine ketones have cleared and blood glucose levels return to the target range. The health care provider should be contacted, and provided there is no medical emergency, the pump manufacturer can also be called to provide technical assistance as mentioned earlier.

In general, infusion sets should be changed every 24 to 72 hours. If blood appears in the tubing, the set should be replaced immediately to avoid potential blocking of insulin delivery. Also, inserting the infusion set before the administration of a bolus reduces the possibility of the needle becoming clogged. Using buffered insulin also helps prevent insulin precipitation and clogging. Insulin aspart (Novolog) has been shown to be more stable for CSII therapy and has a Food and Drug Administration indication for pump use.

■ Hypoglycemia

Patients on CSII are at no greater risk for hypoglycemia than patients using multiple-injection regimens and, as mentioned earlier, pump therapy may in fact reduce the risk for hypoglycemia. Nonetheless, strategies for avoiding hypoglycemia are applicable to any intensive diabetes management program. Therefore, patients and family members should be taught methods of hypoglycemia awareness and how to suspend pump operation in the event of a hypoglycemic episode (see Chapter 13, *Acute Complications*).

■ Skin Infection

Skin infection is one of the more common causes listed for discontinuation of CSII. Most cases of infection have been bacterial, usually *Staphylococcus* or *Streptococcus*. Rarely, the infection may lead to cellulitis or abscess formation requiring surgical debridement. Usually, the infection involves a small area of mild inflammation and tenderness that can be easily treated with antibiotics. These cases often occur in patients who leave the insulin lines in too long (ie, 4 to 6 days).

To avoid infection, the infusion set should be kept clean and dry, and the skin should be cleansed with soap and water before needle insertion. Patients should be instructed to remove moist tape and to clean and dry the area around the needle insertion site. This is especially important during warm weather or in the event of vigorous physical activity.

Most infusion site problems, such as difficulty with needle insertion and skin breakdown, can be resolved by finding the right kind of catheter and tape. Most infusion sets come with self-adhesive tape; however, use of an additional adhesive dressing or surgical tape can help keep the needle in place. The infusion set should not be placed at the belt line or where constrictive clothing might create friction.

The infusion set should be removed every 24 to 72 hours and never be reused. Subsequent infusion sites should be at least 1 inch apart and rotated to a different location. The cannula or needle should be removed immediately in the event of irritation, redness, or inflammation. If any redness persists or worsens, the health care provider should be notified within 24 hours.

Everyday Management

Modern pumps are small enough to be worn during most activities, with the possible exception of physically strenuous athletics. They can be worn on a belt, in a pocket, or clipped to underclothing. During sleep, the pump can be situated on the bed, under pillows, or attached to nightclothes. If the pump is not waterproof, it must be removed, disconnected, held in one hand, or put into a zip-lock bag during showering.

Initiating discussion about sexual activity and pump use is an important aspect of patient education, especially since people often harbor concerns about this topic but are too embarrassed to raise it themselves. The pump may be removed during sexual activity via the quick-release catheter; however, it should be reconnected within an hour. If the pump is not disconnected during sex, it should be checked afterward to ensure that the system is still intact.

Patients may not wish to wear their pumps for certain activities, such as swimming or playing sports, or they may want to take a "vacation" from CSII. The only disadvantage of using fast-acting analogues such as aspart or lispro in pumps is that it significantly shortens the time that a patient can safety disconnect without causing insulinopenia and hyperglycemia. Patients contemplating a prolonged respite from pump use should be advised about the timing and dosing of subcutaneously administered insulin, the scheduling of meals, and the need for continued frequent blood glucose monitoring. The easiest thing to do is to return to the patient's previous regimen used before switching to the pump. Another simple and effective regimen is to switch to insulin glargine (Lantus) for basal insulin and continue insulin lispro (Humalog) and insu-

130

lin aspart (Novolog) before meals using the same doses as used for boluses when wearing the pump. To calculate the dose of Lantus, the patient must determine how much of the daily insulin requirements were given as the basal (total 24-hour usage minus the amount given before meals and snacks).

When switching to Lantus, the first injection should be taken at 5 or 6 PM and continue using the pump until bedtime, then take off the pump. The reason for overlapping this therapy is that Lantus takes a long time to get into the patient's system and if the pump is stopped at the time of taking the initial dose, blood sugar will be excessively high in the morning.

Patient Selection and Education

Beginning CSII involves more than simply changing the mode of insulin delivery. Patients should be educated within the context of a formal program run by a motivated, flexible, and skilled health care team. For example, a dietician should instruct the patient in proper meal planning and carbohydrate counting. A diabetes educator should explain insulin pump management. A psychologist and/or social worker should evaluate motivation, cognitive, and problem-solving skills, financial stability, maturity level, and social support systems. Many patients already on an intensive multiple-injection regimen should have most of the education and skills needed to commit to pump therapy.

Table 9.4 lists characteristics that may help in identifying patients well-suited for CSII. However, it should be remembered that there are no clear-cut criteria. The prevailing concept is that the motivated, relatively stable patient is the best candidate for pump therapy. Yet, another school of thought contends that patients with poorly controlled diabetes who may, in addition, not possess optimal motivation, cognitive

TABLE 9.4 — Characteristics to Consider When Evaluating a Potential Continuous Subcutaneous Insulin Infusion User

Positive Characteristics
- Motivated to perform self-monitoring of blood glucose levels
- Capable of assembling and changing the catheter infusion set
- Clear understanding of self-care, including recognizing and treating hypoglycemia, DKA, infection
- Self-motivated to pursue CSII
- Appropriate awareness of pros and cons of CSII
- Presence of a skilled and enthusiastic health care team
- Able to communicate effectively with the health care team
- Possession of adequate health insurance
- Capable of making simple calculations for carbohydrate counting

Abbreviations: CSII, continuous subcutaneous insulin infusion; DKA, diabetic ketoacidosis.

Adapted from: Lenhard MJ, Reeves GD. *Arch Intern Med.* 2001;161:2297.

skills, or social support could stand to benefit the most from CSII. In the absence of definitive data to clarify these issues, all CSII candidates should undergo an emotional and psychosocial assessment to prevent discontinuation of therapy or misuse of the pump. Some patients may, for example, worry about their perceived lack of physical attractiveness while wearing the pump. Others may feel embarrassed or affronted when strangers inquire about it. Also, while the pump may represent greater self-reliance for many people, it can sometimes evoke feelings of vulnerability or fear of mechanical failure. Patient and family education prior to beginning CSII can help to put such misgivings into perspective or, alternatively, identify individuals who might not do well on the pump.

Special patient populations, such as pregnant women and adolescents, may prefer CSII because of its association with a reduced risk for hypoglycemia and glycemic excursions. Other advantages for pregnant women include increased ease of treating morning sickness and hyperemesis gravidarum, ease of treating the dawn phenomenon that increases during pregnancy, and improved management during the postpartum period when insulin requirements may fluctuate. Nevertheless, initiating pump therapy during pregnancy is not recommended because novice pump users are at greater risk for diabetic ketoacidosis, which would harm the fetus.

The "Untethered" Regimen

Untethered regimen refers to the therapeutic combination of simultaneously using an insulin pump and insulin glargine (Lantus) to improve glycemic excursions and overall control. Insulin glargine (MDI regimen) does have some advantages over pump therapy, especially when a patient is involved in activities that are not pump friendly (eg, swimming, scuba diving). Another advantage of insulin glargine over pump therapy is that there is less concern of sudden, unexpected, and aggravating episodes of severe hyperglycemia and DKA because of infusion-line disruptions. Battery life is not an issue with MDI therapy. However, an MDI regimen cannot provide the ease of bolusing throughout the day before meals and for catch-up doses that pump therapy can offer, as well as the square- and dual-wave bolus features.

To reap the benefits of both insulin pump and MDI therapy, it is possible to split the basal requirements. For example, 75% of the patient's basal requirements can be given as insulin glargine at bedtime and set the basal rate of the pump to give the remaining 25%. A patient whose 24-hour basal requirement is

133

20 units would take 15 units Lantus at bedtime and set the pump to 0.2 units/hour. Temporary and alternate basal rates can also be tailored according the home glucose monitoring results. There is also no concern about sudden and unexpected hyperglycemia that occurs with planned or unplanned disruption of insulin delivery from pump therapy for any reason.

SUGGESTED READING

Boland E. *Teens Pumping It! Insulin Pump Therapy Guide for Adolescents*. Sylmar, Calif: MiniMed Technologies; 1995.

Brink SJ, Stewart C. Insulin pump treatment in insulin-dependent diabetes mellitus. Children, adolescents, and young adults. *JAMA*. 1986;255:617-621.

Fredrickson I, ed. *The Insulin Pump Therapy Book: Insights From the Experts*. Sylmar, Calif; MiniMed Technologies; 1995.

Klingensmith GJ. *Intensive Diabetes Management*. 3rd ed. Alexandria, Va: American Diabetes Association; 2003.

Lenhard MJ, Reeves GD. Continuous subcutaneous insulin infusion: a comprehensive review of insulin pump therapy. *Arch Intern Med*. 2001;161:2293-2300.

Norby D. *Intensive Insulin Therapy Using an Insulin Infusion Pump: A Guide to Developing a Protocol to Implement Insulin Pump Therapy*. Minneapolis, Minn: Disetronic Medical Systems Inc; 1995.

Pickup J, Keen H. Continuous subcutaneous insulin infusion at 25 years: evidence base for the expanding use of insulin pump therapy in type 1 diabetes. *Diabetes Care*. 2002;25:593-598.

Rudoph JW, Hirsch IB. Assessment of therapy with continuous subcutaneous insulin infusion in an academic diabetes clinic. *Endocr Pract*. 2002;8:401-405.

Strowig SM. Initiation and management of insulin pump therapy. *Diabetes Educ*. 1993;19:50-59.

Walsh J, Roberts R. *Pumping Insulin*. 3rd ed. San Diego, Calif: Torrey Pines Press; 2000.

10 Monitoring Glycemic Status

Methods for evaluating glycemic status are integral to any diabetes management program. Results from monitoring are used to assess the efficacy of therapy and to make adjustments in diet, exercise, and medications with the aim of achieving and sustaining individualized treatment objectives. A combination of physician and patient assessment methods is used to obtain the most accurate information about the degree of metabolic control. The metabolic parameters shown in **Table 10.1** are monitored by the health care team during office visits, while patients are responsible for daily self-monitoring of blood glucose (SMBG), recording of blood glucose data, and urine ketone testing.

Monitoring by the Health Care Team

■ Measuring Plasma Glucose Concentrations

Glycemic status is assessed during office visits by review of the patient's SMBG results (see Chapter 11, *Using Blood Glucose Data Technology for Pattern Management*), as well as regular determinations of glycosylated hemoglobin (A1C) and other proteins. Although day-to-day metabolic control is reflected in measurements of plasma glucose concentrations taken with a blood glucose meter, any reading by itself cannot reliably convey the patient's overall metabolic status because:

- It is difficult to know the meaning of a single random or fasting plasma glucose determination.

TABLE 10.1 — Monitoring of Intensive Management Program by the Health Care Team

Primary indicators of overall metabolic control:
- Glycosylated hemoglobin (A1C):
  - Within 1 percentage point above the upper range of normal (<7%)
  - Within 3 SD from the mean
- Frequency and severity of hypoglycemia
- Adequacy of growth and development in children and weight in adults
- Plasma lipid levels
  - Triglyceride level <150 mg/dL
  - HDL cholesterol level >45 mg/dL (>55 in women)
  - LDL cholesterol level <100 mg/dL

Frequency of office visits:
- Daily to weekly at outset of intensive diabetes management program
- Quarterly after initial stage of stabilization

At each visit:
- Check blood glucose monitoring accuracy
- Review blood glucose data
- Discuss issues of diet
- Discuss any issues of ability to follow the intensive management plan
- Measure A1C
- Note body weight, blood pressure, and growth (in children)
- Evaluate problems with hypoglycemia
- Examine sites of insulin administration

Abbreviations: HDL, high-density lipoprotein; LDL, low-density lipoprotein; SD, standard deviation.

Adapted from: American Diabetes Association. *Intensive Diabetes Management*. 3rd ed. Alexandria, Va: American Diabetes Association; 2003:127.

- Random determinations may reflect peak, trough, or values in between because of the wide daily variations in glucose levels.
- The stress of any office visit may result in higher than usual glucose values.
- Some patients may atypically adhere to their treatment regimen or use extra insulin before an office visit, resulting in an uncharacteristically low glucose level.
- The presence of an intercurrent illness at the time of an office visit can also alter blood glucose levels.

However, multiple blood glucose readings recorded over time and evaluated collectively are an essential means of assessing glycemic control and improving the therapeutic regimen. Inaccurate or discrepant results would be revealed by an A1C assay, which reflects the level of glucose control for the preceding 2 to 3 months. In the absence of adequate SMBG data, other corroborating data are needed to evaluate glycemic status, such as symptoms of hypoglycemia or uncontrolled hyperglycemia.

The timing of the measurements has an impact on the significance of the findings:

- A postprandial sample obtained 1 to 2 hours after a patient has eaten is the most sensitive measurement because glucose levels are the highest during this time; total carbohydrate content of the meal will be reflected in this glucose value.
- A preprandial or fasting plasma glucose level reflects how efficiently carbohydrates from a meal have been cleared from the plasma.

■ Measuring Glycosylated Hemoglobin

Assays of HbA_1, HbA_{1C}, and A1C are used extensively to provide an accurate time-integrated measure of glycemic control over the previous 2 to 3 months and to correlate blood glucose levels with patients' SMBG results. Because these assays do not reflect the glucose level at the time a blood sample is tested, measurements of A1C are not useful for making day-to-day adjustments in the treatment regimen.

Glycation refers to a carbohydrate-protein linkage. This irreversible process occurs as glucose in the plasma attaches itself to the hemoglobin component of red blood cells. Because the lifespan of red blood cells is 120 days, A1C assays reflect average blood glucose concentration over that time.

The amount of circulating glucose concentration to which the red cell is exposed influences the amount of A1C. Therefore, the hyperglycemia of diabetes causes an increase in the percentage of A1C in patients with diabetes; HbA_{1C} shows the greatest change, whereas the remaining species are relatively stable.

Levels of HbA_{1C} and HbA_1 correlate best with the degree of metabolic control obtained several months earlier. Regardless of which assay is used, however, certain conditions can interfere with obtaining accurate results:

- False-low concentrations are likely in the presence of conditions that decrease the life of the red blood cell, such as:
  – Hemolytic anemia
  – Bleeding
  – Sickle cell trait
- False-high concentrations are likely in the presence of conditions that increase the lifespan of the red blood cell, eg, lack of a spleen. Other conditions that produce falsely elevated A1Cs include:
  – Uremia
  – High concentrations of fetal hemoglobin
  – High aspirin doses (>10 g/day)
  – High concentrations of ethanol.

Regular monitoring of A1C (eg, every 3 to 6 months) is essential for all patients with diabetes. On a daily basis, patients typically measure capillary blood glucose levels before meals, postprandially, and at bedtime, particularly with intensive insulin regimens in which near-normal glycemia is being actively pursued. Even when preprandial levels seem satisfactory, patients' A1C results often are higher than expected. This finding would not have been evident through glucose measurements alone, and the need for further efforts to control blood glucose would not have been apparent without obtaining an A1C measurement. Home A1C testing is now available (Becton-Dickinson). The patient applies a drop of blood to a reagent card, which is mailed into a central laboratory. The results are then mailed back to the patient.

A disposable test kit for A1C is now available for home testing by patients with diabetes (Metrika).

New devices that are available or soon to be released will have the capability of measuring serum ketones, lipoproteins, microalbumin, and other important clinical values that traditionally could only be obtained by venipuncture or urine collection and measured in a laboratory.

Monitoring by the Patient

All patients with type 1 diabetes must be expected to monitor glycemic control on a daily basis. This monitoring should consist of SMBG, written and/or electronic record-keeping, and, when appropriate, ketone testing (**Table 10.2**).

■ Self-Monitoring of Blood Glucose

Self-evaluation using capillary blood samples has become one of the more important tools for monitoring and improving glycemic control and making adjustments in the therapeutic regimen. SMBG is a

139

TABLE 10.2 — Patient Monitoring During Intensive Diabetes Management

Self-monitoring of blood glucose
- Before each meal
- At bedtime
- 1 to 2 hours after meals (optional)
- Between 2 AM and 4 AM at least weekly
- When symptoms of hypoglycemia occur

Ketone monitoring
- During any illness
- During unexpected or persistent hyperglycemia
- During times of weight loss (intentional or unexpected)
- Daily during pregnancy

Record keeping

Adapted from: American Diabetes Association. *Intensive Diabetes Management*. 3rd ed. Alexandria, Va: American Diabetes Association; 2003:123.

relatively painless procedure that involves pricking the fingertip with a lancet to obtain a drop of blood that is placed on a test strip. Reagents on the test strip contain an enzyme that causes glucose to react with a dye to produce a color change. The color intensity is proportional to the amount of glucose present. The test strip is placed in a small, hand-held meter that quantifies the glucose concentration using reflectance spectrometry. Some test strips can be read visually; other systems measure the electrical current produced by the glucose oxidation reaction to quantify the glucose concentration. Results obtained by SMBG tend to have good agreement with plasma glucose concentrations obtained by clinical laboratory procedures if done properly. Patient techniques tend to be the source of most discrepancies. Typically, plasma venous glucose measurements are within 15% of the results of whole blood capillary glucose determinations.

SMBG is not a goal in itself but rather a means of achieving the goal of normal or near-normal glycemic control. It should be considered an important part of a comprehensive treatment regimen that includes:

- Diabetes education
- Counseling
- Management by a multidisciplinary team of health care providers.

Goals of treatment and thus the reason for performing SMBG must be mutually defined by the patient and health care team. Patients must be motivated and capable of learning the proper techniques of SMBG and committed to applying the results to modify their treatment. Health care providers must be able to discuss SMBG results in a nonjudgmental, helpful way that provides encouragement through open, honest communication and an atmosphere of support.

Reasons for Performing SMBG

The following reasons for performing SMBG have been outlined in a consensus statement by the American Diabetes Association (ADA):

- *To achieve or maintain a specific level of glycemic control*—As evidenced by results of the Diabetes Control and Complications Trial (DCCT) and United Kingdom Prospective Diabetes Study (UKPDS), intensive therapy that is closely monitored using SMBG can help patients achieve near normoglycemia and delay the onset and slow the progression of diabetic complications in type 1 and type 2 diabetes. Therefore, SMBG at least four times daily is essential for evaluating and adjusting insulin doses in patients on intensive insulin regimens.
- *To prevent and detect hypoglycemia*—Hypoglycemia is a major complication of treatment regi-

mens, particularly those involving intensive application of pharmacologic therapy to achieve near normoglycemia. Therefore, appropriately timed SMBG is the only way to detect asymptomatic hypoglycemia so that corrective action (adjusting insulin, diet, and/or exercise) can be taken.

- *To avoid severe hyperglycemia*—Illness and certain drugs that alter insulin secretion (eg, phenytoin, thiazide diuretics) or action (eg, prednisone) can increase the risk of severe hyperglycemia and/or ketoacidosis. SMBG should be initiated or used more frequently in all of these situations to detect hyperglycemia and initiate appropriate intervention.
- *To adjust care in response to lifestyle changes in patients on pharmacologic therapy*—Glucose levels change in response to variations in diet, exercise, and stressful situations. SMBG can help identify patterns of response to planned exercise and daily activity and help modify insulin therapy during times of increased or decreased caloric consumption.

Table 10.3 lists the advantages and disadvantages of SMBG. Far outweighing any possible disadvantage is the inarguable fact that SMBG enables the patient to be involved in self-management and provides immediate feedback regarding the impact of diet, exercise, and insulin on blood glucose levels. Patients who are educated about SMBG, how to use the results, and how to make self-adjustments of insulin doses can achieve better daily glycemic control and have a better sense of self-control and participation in their own care. SMBG also provides worthwhile feedback that the physician and other members of the diabetes health care team can incorporate into ongoing evaluation of

TABLE 10.3 — Advantages and Disadvantages of Self-Monitoring of Blood Glucose

Advantages:
- Accurate, immediate results for detecting hypoglycemia and hyperglycemia
- Day-to-day assessment of glycemic control
- Follow-up information after changes in treatment to enhance accurate adjustments in therapy
- Enhanced patient independence, self-confidence, and participation in their treatment
- Storage of test results

Disadvantages:
- Discomfort of lancing the finger to obtain blood (many meters today have alternate site testing)
- Complexity of some testing procedures, requiring mental acuity and dexterity
- Potential malfunction of equipment that could lead to inaccurate results that may affect treatment decisions
- False results because of inaccurate technique that may affect treatment decisions

10

the treatment regimen. However, health care professionals need to make a point of requesting and reviewing a patient's SMBG data to provide helpful guidance and encouragement.

Recommended Frequency of SMBG

SMBG is critical for all patients who take exogenous insulin, particularly those on intensive insulin regimens. Frequent testing is necessary to fine-tune an insulin regimen to the needs and responses of a given patient. Ideally, SMBG should be performed four to six times per day (before each meal, at bedtime, and occasionally after meals and at 3 AM, which is the approximate time of the early morning glucose nadir). A more intensive SMBG schedule would be a preprandial and 2-hour postprandial measurement and at bedtime, depending on the frequency of insulin dose.

143

SMBG Systems

A combination of factors affect the overall performance of SMBG meters:

- The analytic performance of the meter
- The ability of the user
- The quality of the test strips
- The downloading capacity of home and office computers.

Analytic error can range from 4% to 33%; a goal of future SMBG systems is an analytic error of $\pm$ 5%. User performance is most affected by the quality and extent of training, which currently is hindered by reimbursement policies for diabetes education. Initial and regular assessments of a patient's SMBG technique are necessary to assure accurate results. Patients need to be advised that test strips can be adversely affected by environmental factors. In addition, cautious use of generic test strips is warranted because of the complex process of calibrating test strips to specific meters.

Examples and features of available blood glucose meters are shown in **Table 10.4**. The ADA Consensus Panel advises periodic comparisons between a patient's SMBG system and a sample obtained simultaneously and measured by a referenced laboratory. It is necessary to keep in mind that whole-blood glucose values are generally 15% lower than plasma values.

Advances in Glucose Monitoring

Over the past several years, home glucose monitoring devices have become smaller, faster, and easier to operate with data analysis capabilities (see Chapter 11, *Using Blood Glucose Data Technology for Pattern Management*). Computer-generated data analysis can assist the caregiver and the patient in many different areas, including data collection from blood glucose meters, certain insulin pumps, and other new devices. Computer software programs can also create charts and graphs that reveal trends and patterns in blood glucose values for easier evaluation by the patient and the caregiver. There are many software programs that are not only user-friendly for the patient but are easy to read and analyze by members of the health care team. Several programs can generate one-page summaries of a person's diabetes monitoring data intended for optimal presentation of information. Information typically provided includes the standard day plot, before and after meals, pie graphs, the preceding 14 days in a combination graph format (where diet, exercise, and medication are shown with blood glucose levels) and a glucose line plot. The goal ranges and usual insulin doses are usually printed on the bottom of the page.

Advances in Devices for Blood-Letting

The finger-stick devices used to get a drop of blood for testing from the patient have improved with depth-adjustable and sharp, thin lancets. There is a meter that has the capability of getting blood from areas other than fingertips, such as the forearm, for patient comfort and convenience. Other companies have developed blood-letting devices that can be used on the fingertips and other areas with special attachments to the "finger sticker." Laser technology has also been designed to facilitate blood-letting for these home devices.

Advances in Continuous Glucose Monitoring

The development of devices to allow for frequently measured or real-time glucose values has tremendous implications for achieving near normalization of glucose control while avoiding the most serious complication of intensive glucose management, hypoglycemia. Patient and caregiver education on how to react to frequently obtained values is needed to derive the maximum benefit from this technology.

145

TABLE 10.4 — Selected Blood Glucose Meters and Their Features

Name	Reference	Blood Volume	Test Time	Lancet Size	Test Range	Hematocrit Range (%)	Test Memory	Insulin Memory
Accu-Chek Compact*	Plasma	1 μL	8 sec	28-gauge	10-600 mg/dL	25-65	100 glucose with time and date, average, highest and lowest readings	None
Accu-Chek Advantage*	Plasma	4 μL	26 sec	28-gauge	10-600 mg/dL	20-65	100 glucose with time and date	None
Ascensia DEX[†]	Plasma	3-4 μL	30 sec	28-gauge	10-600 mg/dL	20-60	100 glucose with time and date, 14-day average and time-specific average	None
Ascensia Elite XL[†]	Plasma	3 μL	30 sec	28-gauge	20-600 mg/dL	20-60	120 glucose with time and date	None
BD Latitude[‡]	Plasma	0.3 μL	5 sec	33-gauge	20-600 mg/dL	25-60	250 glucose with time and date, 7-day, 14-day, and time-specific averaging	250 insulin records

							250 insulin records
BD Logic‡	Plasma	0.3 µL	5 sec	33-gauge	20-600 mg/dL	25-60	250 glucose with time and date, 7-day, 14-day, and time-specific averaging	250 insulin records
Freestyle§	Plasma	0.3 µL	15 sec	25-gauge	20-500 mg/dL	0-60	250 glucose with time and date	None
InDuo¶	Plasma	1 µL	5 sec	28-gauge	20-600 mg/dL	30-55	150 glucose with time and date and 14/30-day average	None
OneTouch Ultra¶	Plasma	1 µL	5 sec	28-gauge	20-600 mg/dL	30-55	150 glucose with time and date and 14-day average	None
OneTouch UltraSmart¶	Plasma	1 µL	5 sec	25- or 28-gauge	20-600 mg/dL	30-55	Over 3,000 records in electronic log-book including glucose analysis, exercise, health data, medication, and food	Yes

10

(Continued)

Name	Reference	Blood Volume	Test Time	Lancet Size	Test Range	Hematocrit Range (%)	Test Memory	Insulin Memory
OneTouch Surestep¶	Plasma	10 µL	15-30 sec	28-gauge	0-500 mg/dL	25-60	150 glucose with time and date and 14/30-day average	None
Precision Q.I.D.#	Plasma	3.5 µL	20 sec	28-gauge	20-600 mg/dL	20-70	125 glucose	None
Precision Xtra#	Plasma	3.5 µL	20 sec	30-gauge	20-500 mg/dL	20-70	450 glucose with time and date and 1/2/4-week average	

* Roche: 1-800-858-8072, www.accu-chek.com.

† Bayer: 1-800-348-8100, www.bayercarediabetes.com.

‡ Becton, Dickinson & Co: 1-888-232-2837, www.bddiabetes.com.

§ Therasense: 1-888-522-5226, www.therasense.com.

¶ Lifescan: 1-800-227-8862, www.lifescan.com.

Medisense: 1-800-527-3339, www.medisense.com.

Hirsch IB. *Endocr Pract.* 2004;10:67-76.

The GlucoWatch Automatic Glucose Biographer (Cygnus) has been one promising technology, providing a means for obtaining frequent, automatic, and noninvasive glucose measurements—up to three readings per hour for as long as 12 hours after a single blood glucose measurement for calibration. Clinical studies with the GlucoWatch in controlled laboratory and home environments have demonstrated accuracy and precision, similar to those of currently available invasive home meters. The device utilizes a technique whereby a low-level electric current is passed through the skin between an anode and a cathode. The amount of glucose extracted at the cathode has been previously demonstrated to correlate with blood glucose in diabetic subjects.

There are several other companies currently working on totally noninvasive methods to measure glucose, such as infrared technology and implantable sensors, that are durable and accurate. Invasive frequent–glucose monitoring systems are also being developed. The currently available Medtronic continuous glucose monitoring system is a pager-size device that can measure a patient's glucose value every 5 minutes for up to 72 hours. The glucose oxidase sensor, which is located inside a small needle, is placed in the subcutaneous tissue and discarded when removed. The patient is blinded to the information, however. When returned to the caregiver after 3 days, the stored data can be analyzed for trends. These devices are currently available from physicians who have purchased the monitoring system. Future generations of this sensor will communicate with an external insulin pump and provide real-time data.

■ **Recording Data**

Results of SMBG should be recorded in a log book that is brought to each office visit so the physician can evaluate the effectiveness of the current insulin regimen and determine what, if any, adjustments are needed (**Figure 10**.1). Selected patients should be instructed to apply their SMBG results as the data become available. Making immediate dosage adjustments based on SMBG feedback is evidence of the true benefit of this self-assessment tool. Additionally, many blood glucose meters are capable of storing multiple readings with their corresponding date and time, and also come with companion software for downloading results to a home or office computer. Yet, even patients who take advantage of this technology should keep a written logbook for tracing and correcting lapses in optimal blood glucose control. Chapter 11, *Using Blood Glucose Data Technology for Pattern Management,* describes ways in which patients and physicians can best:

- Analyze and use SMBG data to assess progress toward treatment goals
- Identify blood glucose patterns
- Discern trends that can aid in the formulation of more precise and effective therapeutic regimens.

■ Ketone Monitoring

Ketone monitoring is essential in certain situations to avoid the development of potentially life-threatening diabetic ketoacidosis. Blood or urine ketones should be checked:

- When blood glucose is unexpectedly or repeatedly >240 mg/dL
- During illness
- Daily during pregnancy
- During times of weight loss (intentional or unexpected).

Ketone monitoring can be done using urine monitoring strips or a blood β-hydroxybutyrate–detecting meter, which can also measure blood glucose levels using a different test strip. Many patients prefer urine monitoring over measurement of blood ketones because of the ease of sample collection and the low cost. However, blood ketone monitoring can be better for young children who might not cooperate during urine ketone testing, especially during illness. It is also preferable during a gastrointestinal illness, when slight dehydration may result in concentrated urine, causing the urine ketone value to falsely indicate severe ketonuria.

For patients using an insulin pump, ketonemia or ketonuria, especially when accompanied by hyperglycemia, may signal an interruption of insulin delivery. Patients who are deliberately restricting calorie consumption to lose weight are often on very low doses of insulin to avoid hypoglycemia and therefore should measure ketones regularly. Pregnant women with type 1 diabetes, whose insulin needs may be markedly increased, must also monitor urinary ketones daily.

SUGGESTED READING

10

American Diabetes Association. *Intensive Diabetes Management.* 3rd ed. Alexandria, Va: American Diabetes Association; 2003.

The Diabetes Control and Complications Trial Research Group. The effect of intensive treatment of diabetes on the development and progression of long-term complications in insulin-dependent diabetes mellitus. *N Engl J Med.* 1993;329:977-986.

Edelman SV, Bell JM, Serrano RB, Kelemen D. Home testing of fructosamine improves glycemic control in patients with diabetes. *Endocr Pract.* 2001;7:454-458.

Fleming DR. Accuracy of blood glucose monitoring for patients: what it is and how to achieve it. *Diabetes Educ.* 1994;20:495-500.

Goldstein DE, Little RR, Lorenz RA, et al. Tests of glycemia in diabetes. *Diabetes Care.* 2003;26(suppl 1):S106-S108.

Goldstein DE, Little RR, Lorenz RA, Malone JI, Nathan D, Peterson CM. Tests of glycemia in diabetes. *Diabetes Care.* 1995;18:896-909.

FIGURE 10.1 — Weekly Self-Monitoring Blood Glucose Record Sheet

Name _____

Address _____

City _____

State _____ Zip _____ – _____

SSI #: _____ – _____ – _____

Home PH#: (___) ___ – ___

Work PH#: (___) ___ – ___

Fax #: (___) ___ – ___

Pager #: (___) ___ – ___

INSTRUCTIONS: Record time of day in upper box and glucose readings in lower box.

Day/Date (m/d/y)	AM Breakfast Before	AM Breakfast After	AM INSULIN	Noon	PM Dinner Before	PM Dinner After	PM INSULIN	Comments
SUNDAY __/__/__								
MONDAY __/__/__								
TUESDAY __/__/__								

152

						Weekly Averages
WEDNESDAY __/__/__						
THURSDAY __/__/__						
FRIDAY __/__/__						
SATURDAY __/__/__						

Daily Averages

	SUNDAY	MONDAY	TUESDAY	WEDNESDAY	THURSDAY	FRIDAY	SATURDAY
TIMES OF DAY							
GLUCOSE READINGS							
WEIGHT							

TOTAL UNITS FOR THE WEEK: AM _____ + PM _____ =

10

153

Greyson J. Quality control in patient self-monitoring of blood glucose. *Diabetes Care.* 1993;16:1306-1308.

Harris MI, Cowie CC, Howie LJ. Self-monitoring of blood glucose by adults with diabetes in the United States population. *Diabetes Care.* 1993;16:1116-1123.

Hirsch IB. Blood glucose monitoring technology: translating data into practice. *Endocr Pract.* 2004;10:67-76.

Nettles A. User error in blood glucose monitoring. The National Steering Committee for Quality Assurance Report. *Diabetes Care.* 1993;16:946-948.

Peragallo-Dinko V, ed. *A Core Curriculum for Diabetes Education*, 2nd ed. Chicago, Ill: American Association of Diabetes Educators; 1993:259-279.

Porte D, Sherwin RS. *Ellenberg & Rifkin's Diabetes Mellitus.* 5th ed. Stamford, Conn: Appleton and Lange; 1997.

11 Using Blood Glucose Data Technology for Pattern Management

Pattern management, based on review of blood glucose monitoring data, enables patients with diabetes to make appropriate adjustments in insulin dose, food intake, and/or physical activity so that target metabolic goals may be achieved. Until recently, pattern management depended entirely on the patient's keeping a written logbook detailing blood glucose levels and activity over time. Theoretically, the steps were as follows:

- The patient keeps a record of everything that has occurred since the last visit to the doctor.
- By recording this information, the patient gains insight into the specific factors influencing glycemic control.
- The doctor looks at the logbook, analyzes the entries, and prescribes the ideal treatment or suggests changes.
- The patient's blood glucose levels are better controlled as the result of appropriate treatment.

Unfortunately, this ideal scenario seldom occurs. One reason is that the human brain cannot readily extract complex patterns from the voluminous data contained in a comprehensive logbook. Moreover, the vast majority of patients with diabetes do not monitor blood glucose often enough to evaluate glycemic trends. In fact, one large survey assessing self-monitoring of blood glucose (SMBG) use in the 1990s indicates that only 38% of Americans with diabetes performed SMBG at least once daily; in keeping with a subsequent report that although the number of meter owners rose 10% in the past year, the average number of tests per month decreased among patients in nearly every therapeutic category.

Optimal pattern management is further hampered by the dearth of large-scale observational studies examining how SMBG data may best be used in the clinical setting. In the absence of evidence-based guidelines, the sheer abundance and complexity of information produced by current blood glucose monitoring technology can deter time-pressed clinicians from interpreting the data in a meaningful fashion. Patients in turn may be discouraged from monitoring more frequently, knowing their health care provider is unable or unwilling to translate the results into recommendations that will improve outcomes.

This chapter describes ways in which the traditional logbook can be used in conjunction with blood glucose monitoring technology to improve the quality and efficiency of diabetes care in clinical practice. It is based on the premise that thorough, systematic interpretation of SMBG data is not only feasible in the clinical setting but essential to motivating patient self-management, evaluating progress toward treatment goals, and identifying blood glucose trends that can aid in the formulation of more effective therapy programs.

Logbooks and Memory Meters

Blood glucose meters with memory storage have been available since the late 1980s. The earliest programs for reviewing memory were primitive by today's standards, providing little more than a list of individual glucose measurements and testing times. Adjustments in diet, activity, and pharmacotherapy to normalize blood glucose levels while avoiding severe hypoglycemia were based primarily on information from patient logbooks. Although logbooks remain an integral part of diabetes care today, self-reported data have many shortcomings. For example, patients may add phantom values in logbooks or modify glucose levels that exceed the target range. One study showed that only 23% of logbooks were error-free and less than half contained clinically accurate data.

Currently, almost all of the >20 types of meters on the market may be used in tandem with software programs that allow downloading of blood glucose data (**Table 10.4**). Because these software programs synthesize numerous test results in a wide variety of formats, they are more efficient than logbooks for tracking and modifying glycemic trends. Yet they remain underutilized, largely because many clinicians are wary of the mechanics of integrating this technology into their practice and the perceived commitment of time involved in educating patients about its utility. Focusing on a few of the more practical features offered by today's blood glucose monitoring technology—ie, frequency of testing, blood glucose averages, and standard deviation (SD)—is an effective way for clinicians in almost any office setting to venture beyond the written logbook while avoiding the pitfalls of information overload.

Logistics of Downloading Data in the Office Setting

Computerized downloading of blood glucose data relieves the burden of diabetes care in the clinic by allowing more efficient and focused analysis of available information. A logistic model that works well in the clinic is to assign one or two people to upload meter data and then distribute a printout for viewing by the both the patient and the health care provider. This is done while the patient is waiting, to ensure that there is no disruption of patient flow. In offices not devoted exclusively to patients with diabetes, the added measure of setting up "mini diabetes clinics," whereby certain days or time periods are set aside for diabetic patients, may increase efficiency because personnel familiar with procedures for software downloading can be scheduled accordingly.

During the office visit, the patient and clinician discuss the downloaded data, which provides a "big-picture" perspective that affords pattern recognition not possible with the use of logbooks alone. However, once out-of-target levels and problematic trends are identified, the written logbook may be examined for useful clues to their etiology and correction. The written record can also be used to clarify the appropriate timing of the patterns (clocks on blood glucose meters are often inaccurate). From the patient's perspective, manually writing down blood glucose results draws attention to those outside the target range. Although some patients resist making daily entries in a written logbook, they will usually cooperate when asked to record their blood glucose levels for one week preceding their scheduled visit. Entering insulin doses, exercise, and food intake over the three days prior to the appointment is also helpful in recognizing glycemic patterns.

Because of the wide variety of meters available, diabetes management software that can accept and integrate data from multiple devices is usually more practical than loading numerous individual software programs onto a single office computer. Clinipro (NuMedics Inc, Beaverton, Ore) is one such program that has been used successfully. (Information about software programs that support input from more than one brand of meter may be found at www.mendosa.com.) In all cases, backing up the downloaded data should become part of the office routine.

Interpreting Glucose Downloads

Whereas meter memories provide a limited view of a patient's glycemic profile at any given time—often apart from factors such as diet, exercise, and pharmacologic therapy—accompanying software programs present large volumes of blood glucose data in varying contexts that facilitate pattern management. This information enables the clinician, patient, and other members of the management team to set goals, monitor progress from one visit to another, identify problems, and evaluate interventions.

Software programs differ in terms of their statistical and graphic formats. The typical data management system will provide an "electronic logbook" listing blood glucose readings by date and time. Many offer statistical summaries, including:

- Average blood glucose reading and average number of blood glucose tests per day
- Proportion of readings above, below, and within the target range
- Frequency of blood glucose readings by day of the week and by time period within a given day
- SD indicating glycemic variability over specified time periods.

The information is presented in tables as well as multicolor visual displays (eg, pie charts, histograms, and modal day/week graphs that plot blood glucose readings against a single 24-hour or 7-day period). More sophisticated programs correlate glucose levels with insulin types and dosages, food intake, and exercise. Some include companion programs that run on personal digital assistant (PDA) systems.

Realistically, few patients or clinicians will be sufficiently motivated to avail themselves of all of these features. However, regular review of certain informa-

11

tion, ie, frequency of testing, blood glucose averages, and SD, provides important insights into helping patients improve and/or maintain glycemic control.

■ Frequency of Testing

When considering frequency of testing, it is necessary to ask this key question: Is the frequency sufficient at each time of day to achieve optimal glycemic control? Meter downloads display in various ways, both numerically and graphically, the number of tests per day and frequency of testing at particular times of the day. Physicians should review this information with the patient to identify overall trends and delineate areas in need of improvement. This process often encourages patients to test more frequently because they know the data generated by the computer will objectively mirror their effort.

■ Averages

The most potentially revealing question when reviewing averages is: Does the average match the A1C and, if not, why is there a discrepancy? Averages of blood glucose levels provide a quick, though superficial, impression of whether the patient has been maintaining glycemic levels within the target range. However, closer scrutiny is required to ascertain glycemic variability, an often overlooked component of successful pattern management. When a patient shows average fasting blood glucose levels within the target range but a high A1C, it is likely that the patient is experiencing hyperglycemic intervals not captured by the SMBG. Identifying the circumstances behind these episodes will often result in more refined analyses of blood glucose trends and thus more targeted recommendations for treatment.

It should be noted that when determining averages for a specific time period, such as lunch or dinner, it may be necessary to manually program time frames to reflect the actual time of eating if outside the normal parameters. When using software at home, this manual adjustment may be implemented during setup of the program by the patient. In the clinic, however, customizing mealtimes may be cumbersome, especially if meter downloading is done by clinic support staff rather than the health care provider in charge of reviewing the data.

■ Standard Deviation

SD of blood glucose values, or the square root of the variance, indicates whether glycemia is being controlled consistently or with drastic swings indicative of suboptimal disease management. It is thus important to ask: Does the degree of glycemic variability ensure safe glycemic control? Following is a relatively easy formula for interpreting the significance of SD: twice the SD should be less than the average blood glucose level (SD $\times$ 2 < average level). This formula may be carried out by quick inspection of the software printout; however, it signifies only an initial goal for glycemic variability. Even more desirable would be an average exceeding three times the SD (SD $\times$ 3 < average level), though this standard is admittedly unrealistic for the typical patient receiving insulin. In our observation, the higher the SD, the lower the secretion of endogenous insulin; and as a rule, patients with type 1 diabetes exhibit higher SD than those with type 2 disease. Although never formally studied, the fasting average and SD appear to be good indicators of endogenous insulin secretion.

The SD has other uses. A high SD is associated with poor coordination of caloric intake and administration of prandial insulin, a problem especially common among teenagers who tend to snack erratically. Other possible causes of high SD include missed or late injections, gastroparesis, and erratic insulin absorption.

Many blood glucose software programs record SD at different times of day, which can be particularly useful in identifying problems and adjusting therapy. For example, a prebreakfast blood glucose average of 125 mg/dL with an SD of 45 mg/dL indicates good glycemic control, yet the same average at bedtime with an SD of 90 mg/dL raises suspicion of significant hyperglycemia or hypoglycemia, likely resulting from a mismatching of insulin and carbohydrates at dinner. This pattern is common and frequently warrants a subsequent appointment to review carbohydrate counting with a nutritionist. Also, it is important to note that neither averages nor SD can be reliably interpreted for a given time of day if the number of readings is too low. For instance, a high average and SD based on only three readings should be considered inconclusive. Although there are no studies to assist the clinician as to the minimum number of tests required, five to ten readings are usually enough to ensure valid results.

■ Pie Charts and Histograms

Pie charts and histograms are often favored by patients because they are easy to comprehend at a glance. Colorful representations of the data discussed, in addition to such information as the number of blood glucose levels above, below, or within the target range, provide tangible feedback that can be motivating for some patients. Additionally, in contrast to written data from logbooks, blood glucose downloading offers objective reference points for discussion, which in our experience results in more meaningful and efficient communication between the patient and the diabetes care team.

Case Presentations

- **Case #1 — A 34-year-old woman with type 1 diabetes on continuous subcutaneous insulin infusion (CSII)**

This motivated patient lives alone and travels frequently on business. She has been on CSII approximately 1 year, a choice she made to accommodate her hectic schedule. She checks her blood glucose five times per day and her A1C is 7.3%. Her meter download showed the following data for the month prior to her clinic visit:

	Night	5 AM-9 AM	9 AM-11 AM	11 AM-2 PM	2 PM-4 PM	4 PM-8 PM	8 PM-10 PM	10 PM-12 PM	Overall
Mean (mg/dL)	134	**170**	**109**	137	**143**	166	**110**	133	**137**
SD	49	**61**	**57**	52	**87**	62	**55**	51	**63**

Although this patient's overall average and SD of 137 and 63 are acceptable ($63 \times 2 = 126$), a closer look at the time-specific averages and SD reveals important concerns. First, her morning average is too high, suggesting that her basal insulin dose overnight is too low. Next, her midmorning average of 109 with an SD of 57 suggests she is taking too much morning insulin. More extensive history is required to understand whether this is the result of too much insulin at breakfast, too much for the correction dose in response to the morning hyperglycemia, or perhaps too much morning basal insulin. Similarly, the after-lunch and after-dinner SD are too high relative to the averages, which although within target, suggest frequent hypoglycemia because of the large glycemic variation. Upon further questioning, the patient revealed that she had increased her prandial insulin doses far above the recommendation at the last clinic visit to ensure better glycemic control while traveling, which explained the frequent episodes of postprandial hypoglycemia.

163

She had been unaware of this trend prior to review of the downloaded logbook at our clinic. At the conclusion of her appointment, she agreed to reduce mealtime insulin doses to better match carbohydrate intake.

- ■ **Case #2 — An 18-year-old girl with type 1 diabetes reporting recent severe episode of hypoglycemia**

The scattered logbook entries of this patient, typical of many teenagers, show numerous above-target blood glucose levels, which were confirmed by the meter download obtained during her office visit. She mentioned that her after-school job at a fast-food restaurant offered many opportunities for snacking and that she tended to "graze" throughout the day rather than eat well-balanced regular meals. Her insulin regimen consisted of relatively large doses of insulin glargine at bedtime (40 to 45 U) and insulin lispro before meals. However, erratic eating habits and self-consciousness about injecting during the day often caused her to misjudge the timing of her premeal injections or to skip them altogether. Her A1C was 7.9%, and she reported several episodes of mid-evening hypoglycemia, one of which was severe enough to require intervention by her mother. Her blood glucose download showed the following:

	Night	5 AM-9 AM	9 AM-11 AM	11 AM-2 PM	2 PM-4 PM	4 PM-8 PM	8 PM-10 PM	10 PM-12 PM	Overall
Mean (mg/dL)	263	202	252	201	186	206	**162**	199	**201**
SD	162	65	106	102	119	107	**127**	116	**108**

The high SD and mean overall blood glucose level indicate the patient's inability to consistently adhere to her current regimen. The only mean within the target range occurred during the evening, with the accompanying high SD marking the hypoglycemic event. The patient explained that she seldom had an appetite for dinner after arriving home from work, which accounted

164

for the high incidence of hypoglycemia in the early evening. However, the average frequency of 5.6 tests per day showed her willingness to adopt positive self-management practices. The physician explained that insulin glargine used as a basal insulin obviated the need for frequent snacking, and he recommended a more consistent meal schedule, including dinner. Yet, understanding the social and practical pressures faced by this busy teen, he substituted the lunchtime injection of lispro with an injection of regular insulin to cover her mid-afternoon snacking. This compromise satisfied the patient, who agreed to count carbohydrates more vigilantly, especially during the evening, to avert future episodes of hypoglycemia.

Summary

Several important conclusions from these cases should be emphasized. First, the use of means and SD does not follow all of the rules of classical statistics. It would be rare to find blood glucose data normally distributed, and the formula SD × 2 < average level is not helpful when the average is low. It is difficult to cite an exact average blood glucose level below which this formula does not apply, but take the patient who has 25 bedtime blood glucose levels with an average of 89 and an SD of 39. Although this patient meets the standard for the SD × 2 < average level, in reviewing the individual numbers, 11 of these numbers are <60 mg/dL. Similarly, when the average is extremely high, the SD becomes less meaningful since the average is so far from target.

Outliers are also an important issue, particularly when fewer data points are captured. They need to be interpreted individually, and may make drawing conclusions from the mean and SD difficult. It should therefore be noted that while the mean and SD are quite useful in blood glucose data management, certain caveats need to be appreciated. Glucose downloads should, ideally, be used in conjunction with the written logbook, despite the fact that many patients find the latter tedious to maintain on a long-term basis. Clearly, more research in this area is required.

SUGGESTED READING

American Diabetes Association. Self-monitoring of blood glucose (Consensus Statement). *Diabetes Care*. 1997;20:S62-S64.

American Diabetes Association. Standards of medical care in diabetes. *Diabetes Care*. 2005;28(suppl 1):S4-S36.

American Diabetes Association. Tests of glycemia in diabetes. *Diabetes Care*. 2002;25:S97-S99.

Benjamin EM. Self-monitoring of blood glucose: the basics. *Clinical Diabetes*. 2002;20:45-47.

Bloomgarden ZT. Treatment issues in type 1 diabetes. *Diabetes Care*. 2002;25:230-236.

Evans JM, Newton RW, Ruta DM, MacDonald TM, Stevenson RJ, Morris AD. Frequency of blood glucose monitoring in relation to glycemic control: observational study with diabetes database. *BMJ*. 1999;319:83-86.

Gonder-Frederick LA, Julian DM, Cox DJ, Clarke WL, Carter WR. Self-measurement of blood glucose. Accuracy of self-reported data and adherence to recommended regimen. *Diabetes Care*. 1988;11:579-585.

Hirsch IB. Blood glucose monitoring technology: translating data into practice. *Endocr Pract*. 2004;10:67-76.

Mazze RS, Shamoon H, Pasmantier R, et al. Reliability of blood glucose monitoring by patients with diabetes mellitus. *Am J Med*. 1984;77:211-217.

Saaddine JB, Engelgau MM, Beckles GL, Gregg EW, Thompson TJ, Narayan KM. A diabetes report card for the United States: quality of care in the 1990s. *Ann Intern Med*. 2002;136:565-574.

Skyler JS, Lasky IA, Skyler DL, Robertson EG, Mintz DH. Home blood glucose monitoring as an aid in diabetes management. *Diabetes Care*. 1978;1:150-157.

Ziegler O, Kolopp M, Got I, Genton P, Debry G, Drouin P. Reliability of self-monitoring of blood glucose by CSII-treated patients with type 1 diabetes. *Diabetes Care*. 1989;12:184-188.

11

12 Pramlintide Therapy

The discovery of insulin over 80 years ago is one of the great success stories in the history of modern medicine. Even today, insulin remains the most potent hypoglycemic agent in our therapeutic armamentarium and continues to save millions of lives around the world. Advances in its pharmacology and delivery, such as the development of rapid-acting and long-acting insulin analogs, have increased the efficacy, safety, and convenience of its use in intensive therapy regimens.

Despite this considerable progress, however, relatively few insulin-treated patients with type 1 diabetes manage to achieve optimal glycemic control (see Chapter 6, *Glycemic Goals*). Although this "failure" can be attributed in part to socioeconomic, motivational, and educational factors, several clinical shortcomings of subcutaneously administered insulin therapy impede the safe achievement of near-normal glycemia (**Table 12.1**).

Arguably, the greatest deterrents to the use of intensive insulin regimens are hypoglycemia, the fear of hypoglycemia, and the need for frequent fine-tuning of insulin doses on a day-to-day basis (see Chapter 8, *Multiple-Component Insulin Regimens*). Additionally, current insulin formulations and methods of delivery fail to duplicate insulin action of healthy individuals, especially during the postprandial period when, normally, there is a rapid surge of insulin into the portal vein. Weight gain is another key deterrent to the pursuit of normoglycemia with insulin.

While insulin remains the mainstay of therapy for people with type 1 diabetes, the quest for more physiologic and thus more effective approaches to treatment

TABLE 12.1 — Clinical Barriers Associated With Insulin Therapy

Clinical Barrier	Comments
Increased risk of hypoglycemia	• Risk increases exponentially as patients approach normoglycemia • Risk sustained over years
Failure to normalize postprandial glucose excursion	• Insulin replacement is still not physiologic (subcutaneous vs portal) • Rapid-acting insulin analogues still cannot restore postprandial normoglycemia • Insulin is only one of the hormonal regulators of postprandial glucose homeostasis
Excessive diurnal glucose fluctuations	• Make it difficult for patients to predict glucose levels and adjust insulin therapy
Excessive weight gain	• Underappreciated in patients with type 1 diabetes • Cosmetic concern of many patients • Negative effects on lipids and blood pressure

Adapted from: Edelman SV, Weyer C. *Diabetes Technol Ther*. 2002;4:175-189.

has prompted investigation of other glucoregulatory hormones. These include the β-cell hormone amylin, the α-cell hormone glucagon, and numerous gut-derived hormones, such as the incretins glucagon-like polypeptide-1 (GLP-1) and gastric inhibitory peptide (GIP). Because the effects of some, if not all, of these hormones are dysregulated in people with diabetes, many researchers now believe that achieving glucose homeostasis requires a multipronged effort involving more than replacement of insulin alone. Therefore, therapies have been developed that address these hormonal imbalances. Along these lines, replacing the function of both pancreatic β-cell hormones, amylin and insulin, may afford more complete restoration of the physiology of glucose control. The synthetic human amylin analog, pramlintide, which retains the desired biologic activities of human amylin but has superior stability and solubility, represents an important new potential therapeutic option for patients with diabetes. Pramlintide acetate injection (Symlin) was approved by the Food and Drug Administration (FDA) in March 2005 as an adjunct treatment for patients with type 1 and type 2 diabetes who use mealtime insulin therapy and who have failed to achieve desired glucose control despite optimal insulin therapy.

The New Paradigm: Addressing Glucose Appearance and Disappearance

Insulin controls postprandial glucose by two major mechanisms. First, it promotes the uptake of glucose into insulin-sensitive peripheral tissues. Second, it inhibits hepatic glucose output by exerting direct and indirect effects on the liver, including suppression of glucagon secretion. Because these mechanisms of insulin action have been the focal point in treating type 1 diabetes, discussion of the physiology of glycemic regulation has, by extension, emphasized the importance of glucose disposal or disappearance.

In 1987, another pancreatic β-cell hormone, amylin, which is coproduced, costored, and cosecreted with insulin in response to meals, was reported. In healthy individuals, amylin secretion follows the same pattern as insulin: continuous basal secretion with a sharp increase in secretion in response to nutrient uptake (**Figure 12.1**). Amylin is packaged together with insulin in the β-cell granules and, like insulin, is ab-

171

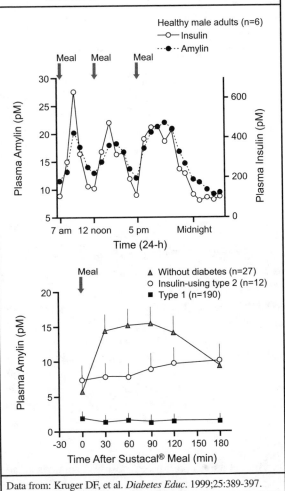

FIGURE 12.1 — Amylin: Co-secreted With Insulin and Deficient in Diabetes

Data from: Kruger DF, et al. *Diabetes Educ*. 1999;25:389-397.

sent or minimally present in people with type 1 diabetes. However, whereas insulin primarily stimulates the disappearance of glucose from plasma, amylin inhibits its appearance through a variety of mechanisms, all of which are thought to be mediated via the central nervous system (**Figure 12**.2):

- Pramlintide slows gastric emptying, ie, the rate of at which food is released from the stomach to the small intestine.
- Pramlintide suppresses glucagon secretion, which leads to suppression of endogenous glucose output from the liver.
- Pramlintide regulates food intake due to centrally-mediated modulation of appetite.

Amylin and insulin work together to regulate glucose appearance and disappearance in a balanced manner. When that regulation is disrupted, as is the case with diabetes, it is only reasonable to assume that optimal therapy cannot be achieved using only one peptide or the other. With the development of pramlintide, a more comprehensive approach to therapy becomes feasible.

12

Mechanisms of Action of Pramlintide

■ Slowing of Gastric Emptying

In healthy individuals, amylin modulates the rate of gastric emptying, most likely via the vagus nerve, to regulate the inflow of nutrients into the small intestine and thereby reduce the postprandial rise in glucose. It is interesting that the rate of gastric emptying is frequently accelerated in people with diabetes. This may be due to amylin deficiency and when pramlintide is administered, there is a slowing in the rate of gastric emptying. In one study, diabetic rats treated with insulin alone were observed to have a markedly accelerated rate of gastric emptying compared with non-

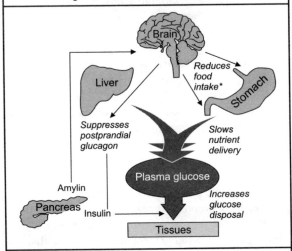

FIGURE 12.2 — Proposed Model of Amylin and Insulin Action in Postprandial Glucose Homeostasis

Insulin is the major hormonal regulator of glucose disposal. Preclinical and clinical studies indicate that amylin complements the effects of insulin by regulating the rate of glucose inflow to the bloodstream.

* Reported in rodents.

Edelman SV, Weyer C. *Diabetes Technol Ther*. 2002;4:180.

diabetic rats, but when rat amylin was administered to both diabetic and nondiabetic rats, a slowing of gastric emptying took place in both groups. Furthermore, comparison of the rates of gastric emptying in rodents given amylin, GLP-1, CCK-8, GIP, glucagon, or pancreatic polypeptide showed that three of the peptides — amylin, GLP-1, and CCK-8 — dose dependently retarded gastric emptying, although the effect of amylin was 15-fold more potent than that of GLP-1 and 20-fold more potent than CCK-8.

Pramlintide administered to patients with type 1 diabetes was found to slow the rate of nutrient delivery from the stomach to the small intestine following intake of both solid and liquid meals. In clinical studies, the half gastric emptying time was extended by approximately 90 minutes (**Figure 12.3**). Thus pramlintide modulates the inflow of glucose into the circulation after meals while still allowing complete emptying of the stomach between meals.

■ Postprandial Glucagon Suppression

Glucagon, secreted from pancreatic α-cells, is a key catabolic hormone that stimulates the release of hepatic glucose reserves during fasting and pro-

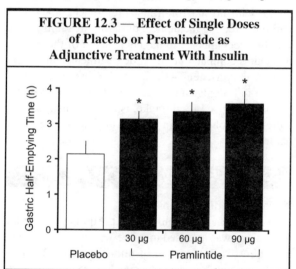

FIGURE 12.3 — Effect of Single Doses of Placebo or Pramlintide as Adjunctive Treatment With Insulin

Effect of single doses of placebo or pramlintide (30, 60, or 90 µg) as adjunctive treatment with insulin on the mean time (+SE) to half gastric emptying of the solid component of a meal determined in a four-way crossover study in 11 men with uncomplicated type 1 diabetes receiving insulin treatment.

Edelman SV, Weyer C. *Diabetes Technol Ther*. 2002;4:183.

tects against hypoglycemia. Inappropriate hypersecretion of glucagon, leading to inadequate suppression of hepatic glucose release at mealtime, contributes to postprandial hyperglycemia in patients with type 1 and type 2 diabetes. Pramlintide helps inhibit glucose appearance in the circulation by suppressing inappropriate glucagon secretion most likely via the parasympathetic nervous system.

■ Regulation of Food Intake

A recent study specifically designed to assess the effects of pramlintide on satiety has shown that pramlintide administered as a single preprandial injection increased levels of satiety leading to reduced food intake with no macronutrient preferences noted and without affecting mean meal duration. In addition, the satiety effect appears to be independent of the nausea that can accompany pramlintide treatment. This information is consistent with the anorexigenic effect of amylin in rodents and suggests that increased satiety, and thus reduced food intake, is a mechanism for the weight loss observed in long-term pramlintide clinical trials.

Clinical Efficacy

■ Postprandial Glucose

The effect of pramlintide on postprandial glucose excursions was assessed in a five-way crossover study in patients with type 1 or insulin-using type 2 diabetes. Following four separate standardized meals, each subject received pramlintide at different times relative to the meal (–15, 0, +15, and +30 minutes), and on one occasion, they received placebo 15 minutes before the meal. Three groups of patients were assessed: type 2 subjects using insulin lispro and type 1 subjects using insulin lispro or human regular insulin. Insulin lispro was administered immediately before meals and human regular insulin was administered 30 minutes before meals. The glucose-lowering effects of pramlintide were greatest when it was administered immediately prior to the meal. Results from this study confirmed that pramlintide, as an adjunct to mealtime insulin therapy, significantly reduced postprandial glucose excursions compared with insulin therapy alone (**Figure 12.4**). Pramlintide achieved its effects with an average reduction in mealtime insulin dose of approximately 30%.

In an open-label study in a clinical setting, 6 months of pramlintide treatment significantly reduced postprandial glucose excursions as assessed by self-monitored 7-point glucose profiles in patients with type 1 and type 2 diabetes (**Figure 12.5**).

■ Long-Term Glycemic Control With Pramlintide

Several long-term clinical trials have shown the benefit of adding pramlintide to an existing regimen of insulin therapy to improve glycemic control. In two representative 1-year trials in patients with type 1 and insulin-requiring type 2 diabetes, pramlintide treatment resulted in significantly reduced glycosylated hemoglobin (A1C) levels from baseline compared with placebo. Moreover, the proportion of patients who were able to achieve the American Diabetes Association (ADA) glycemic target (A1C <7%) was 2-fold to 3-fold greater in pramlintide-treated patients (**Figure 12.6**). Notably, in both type 1 and insulin-requiring type 2 diabetes, the reduction in A1C observed with pramlintide also occurred in patients who were approaching the ADA glycemic targets upon study entry, providing evidence that the use of pramlintide in addition to insulin is effective for facilitating glycemic improvement beyond that achievable with insulin

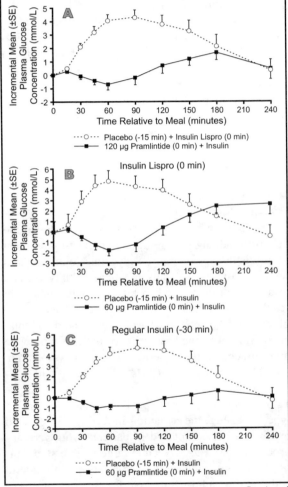

FIGURE 12.4 — Postprandial Glucose Profiles in Subjects With Type 1 and Type 2 Diabetes Relative to a Standard Meal

Continued

178

Postprandial glucose profiles in subjects with *(A)* type 2 diabetes following injections of insulin lispro *(B)* type 1 diabetes following injections of insulin lispro and *(C)* type 1 diabetes following injections of regular insulin plus either placebo (at -15 min) or pramlintide (at 0 min) relative to a standard meal.

Adapted from: *(A)* Maggs DG, et al. *Diabetes Metab Res Rev.* 2004;20:55-60. *(B and C)* Weyer C, et al. *Diabetes Care.* 2003;26:3074-3079.

alone. This improvement was not accompanied by weight gain and, in fact, was associated with a reduction in body weight compared with placebo.

■ Sustained Weight Loss Effects of Pramlintide

Clinical studies have shown that improved glycemic control in pramlintide-treated patients was not accompanied by increased body weight. In fact, the greater reduction in A1C with pramlintide compared with placebo has been associated with a sustained and statistically significant reduction in body weight (**Figure 12.7**). Although the mechanism responsible for this weight loss has not been fully studied in humans, the finding is consistent with the short-term effects of amylin in the regulation of food intake and body fat reserves observed in animal models.

The pooled data from the pivotal trials for pramlintide in type 1 and insulin-requiring type 2 diabetes for A1C reduction, insulin requirements, and weight loss are presented in **Figure 12.8** and **Figure 12.9**. Patients on pramlintide significantly improved their overall glycemic control while losing weight and without a statistically significant increase in their insulin doses. This combination of benefits has not been observed with insulin or any oral antidiabetic agents approved for use.

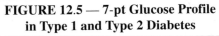

FIGURE 12.5 — 7-pt Glucose Profile in Type 1 and Type 2 Diabetes

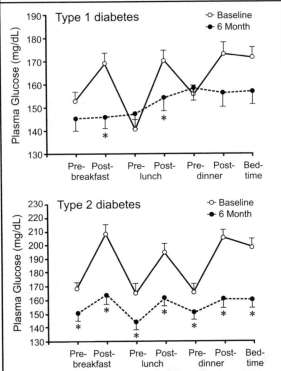

After 6 months of pramlintide therapy as an adjunct to mealtime insulin, postprandial glucose excursions and glucose fluctuations throughout the day were reduced in patients with type 1 and patients with type 2 diabetes.

* $P < 0.05$.

Guthrie R, et al. 65th Annual Scientific Sessions of the American Diabetes Assocation; 2005; Karl D, et al. 65th Annual Scientific Sessions of the American Diabetes Association; 2005.

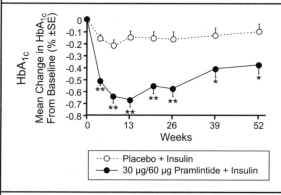

FIGURE 12.6 — Mean Changes From Baseline in HbA$_{1C}$ for Patients With Type 1 Diabetes: Placebo + Insulin vs Pramlintide + Insulin

Mean changes (±SE) from baseline in HbA$_{1c}$ for patients with type 1 diabetes treated with placebo + insulin or pramlintide + insulin. Statistical significance is denoted by * (P <0.05) and ** (P <0.001). Addition of pramlintide to existing insulin therapy led to significant and sustained reduction in HbA$_{1c}$.

Edelman SV, Weyer C. *Diabetes Technol Ther*. 2002;4:184.

12

■ Tolerability

Pramlintide treatment has been shown to be well-tolerated in patients with diabetes. No evidence of cardiac, hepatic, or renal toxicity, changes in serum lipids, or clinically relevant changes in laboratory parameters, vital signs, electrocardiograms, or abnormal findings upon physical examinations have been observed. The most commonly reported adverse events other than hypoglycemia were gastrointestinal (GI) in nature and included nausea, anorexia, and vomiting.

Nausea occurred more frequently in patients with type 1 diabetes than in those with type 2 diabetes. In type 1 diabetes, it occurred in approximately 48% of patients during the clinical development program, was

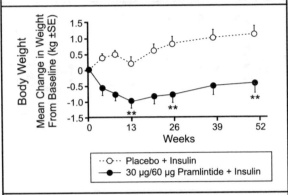

FIGURE 12.7 — Mean Changes From Baseline in Body Weight for Patients With Type 1 Diabetes: Placebo + Insulin vs Pramlintide + Insulin

Mean changes (±SE) from baseline in body weight for patients with type 1 diabetes treated with placebo + insulin or pramlintide + insulin. Statistical significance is denoted by * (P <0.05) and ** (P <0.001). Addition of pramlintide to existing insulin therapy led to significant and sustained reductions in body weight.

Edelman SV, Weyer C. *Diabetes Technol Ther*. 2002;4:184.

generally mild to moderate in intensity, occurred early in the course of therapy and generally resolved over time. Slow titration of pramlintide has been shown to be effective in the management of these GI side effects.

■ Hypoglycemia

Pramlintide has been associated with an increased risk of insulin-induced severe hypoglycemia, particularly in patients with type 1 diabetes. When severe hypoglycemia associated with pramlintide occurs, it is usually seen within the first 3 hours after pramlintide injection.

It should be emphasized that the addition of any antihyperglycemic agent to a patient's current insulin therapy has the potential to increase the risk of hypoglycemia, particularly at the start of therapy. In the long-term pivotal studies in patients with type 1 and insulin-requiring type 2 diabetes where full-dose pramlintide was added to existing insulin regimens in a double-blind fashion without titration, it was observed that the severe hypoglycemia event rate during the first 4 weeks of therapy was greater in the pramlintide group compared with placebo. In a more recent study in patients with type 1 diabetes, it was shown that this risk was short-term and manageable with adequate glucose monitoring, a proactive reduction of premeal insulin doses at initiation of pramlintide, and gradual upward titration of pramlintide dose during its initiation. Based on studies such as this, the recommendation to reduce mealtime insulin by 50% emerged as the most prudent approach to initiating pramlintide therapy while minimizing the risk of insulin-induced hypoglycemia.

An important feature of pramlintide is that its glucose-lowering effects are overcome in the presence of hypoglycemia. One study in patients with type 1 diabetes and another in healthy nondiabetic subjects confirmed preclinical findings that suppression of glucagon by pramlintide is overridden in response to insulin-induced hypoglycemia. Furthermore, insulin clamp studies in subjects with type 1 diabetes have shown that pramlintide, when used as adjunctive therapy to insulin, has no independent effect on the response to hypoglycemia.

■ Pramlintide Widens the Therapeutic Window of Insulin

When insulin is used alone to treat type 1 diabetes and many individuals with insulin-requiring type 2 diabetes, it has a very narrow therapeutic window

183

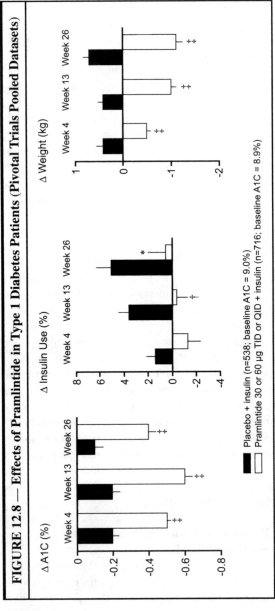

FIGURE 12.8 — Effects of Pramlintide in Type 1 Diabetes Patients (Pivotal Trials Pooled Datasets)

Placebo + insulin (n=538; baseline A1C = 9.0%)
Pramlintide 30 or 60 µg TID or QID + insulin (n=716; baseline A1C = 8.9%)

Abbreviations: A1C, glycosylated hemoglobin; ITT, insulin tolerance test; SE, standard error.

Pivotals 137-112, 137-117, 137-121.

* P <0.05.
† P <0.01.
‡ P <0.0001; ITT population, mean (SE) change from baseline.

Ratner R, et al. *Diabetic Med.* 2004;21:1204-1212; Whitehouse FW, et al. *Diabetes Care.* 2002;25:724-730; Symlin Prescribing Information, 2005.

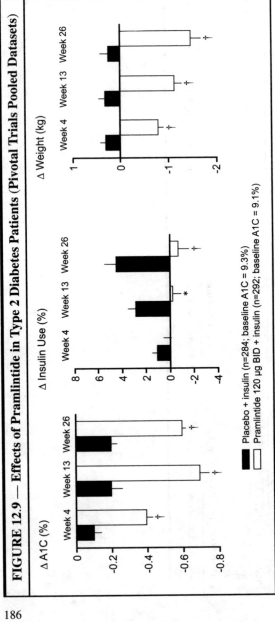

FIGURE 12.9 — Effects of Pramlintide in Type 2 Diabetes Patients (Pivotal Trials Pooled Datasets)

Placebo + insulin (n=284; baseline A1C = 9.3%)

Pramlintide 120 µg BID + insulin (n=292; baseline A1C = 9.1%)

Abbreviations: A1C, glycosylated hemoglobin; ITT, insulin tolerance test; SE, standard error.

Pivotals 137-122, 137-123.

* P <0.01.
† P <0.0001.

Hollander RE, et al. *Diabetes Care.* 2003;26:784-790; Ratner RE, et al. *Diabetes Technol Ther.* 2002;4:51-61; Symlin Prescribing Information, 2005.

12

(**Figure 12.10**). If the dose is too low, hyperglycemia ensues; if too much insulin is given, hypoglycemia occurs. There is not much room for error, especially in people with insulin-sensitive type 1 diabetes. Thus pramlintide addresses the issue of inhibiting excessive glucose appearance, thereby reducing the amount of premeal fast-acting insulin required, and the risk of postprandial hyperglycemia and delayed hypoglycemia are reduced. Pramlintide widens the therapeutic window of insulin. After the appropriate uptitration of pramlintide in conjunction with the lower required dose of premeal insulin, the patient should experience reduced day-to-day glucose fluctuations and less postprandial hyperglycemia and less insulin-induced hypoglycemia.

Dosing of Pramlintide

Pramlintide is available in vials and is injected using a U-100 insulin syringe (a 0.3-cc syringe is recommended). Pramlintide should always be administered in a separate syringe and at a distinct injection site more than two inches away from concomitant in-

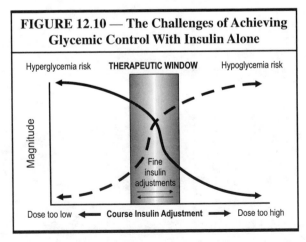

FIGURE 12.10 — The Challenges of Achieving Glycemic Control With Insulin Alone

Hyperglycemia risk   THERAPEUTIC WINDOW   Hypoglycemia risk

Magnitude

Fine insulin adjustments

Dose too low ◄— **Course Insulin Adjustment** —► Dose too high

sulin injections. All patients should reduce premeal insulin by 30% to 50% to lessen the risk of insulin-induced hypoglycemia; monitor blood glucose frequently; and contact their health care provider if symptoms of nausea and/or hypoglycemia are severe or unusually persistent and when the dosage of pramlintide or insulin is changed. Dosing differs depending on whether the patient has type 1 or type 2 diabetes and the general guidelines are:

- **Patients with type 1 diabetes**:
  - Initiate pramlintide at 15 μg taken immediately prior to major meals
  - Titrate pramlintide upward in 15-μg increments when no clinically significant nausea has occurred for at least 3 days at each dose. If significant nausea occurs at the 45- or 60-μg dose decrease the dose to 30 μg. If the 30-μg dose is not tolerated discontinuation of pramlintide should be considered.
  - Optimize insulin to achieve glycemic targets once the maintenance dose of pramlintide is reached and blood glucose concentrations are stable
- **Patients with type 2 diabetes:**
  - Initiate pramlintide at 60 μg taken immediately prior to major meals
  - Titrate pramlintide to 120 μg after 3 to 7 days with no clinically significant nausea
  - Optimize insulin to achieve glycemic targets once the maintenance dose of pramlintide is reached and blood glucose concentrations are stable.

Since pramlintide is prescribed in μg and dosed using an insulin syringe, knowing the conversion from μg to units is important (**Table 12.2**).

TABLE 12.2 — Conversion of Pramlintide Dose to Insulin Unit Equivalents		
Pramlintide Dosage Prescribed (μg)	Increment Using a U-100 Syringe (Units)	Volume (cc or mL)
15	2-1/2	0.025
30	5	0.050
45	7-1/2	0.075
60	10	0.100
120	20	0.200

Practical Tips for Patients on Pramlintide

■ Start With a Low Dose and Titrate Slowly

Pramlintide can cause nausea, anorexia, and vomiting, especially in type 1 diabetes. It is extremely important not to rush the dose titration. In patients with type 1 diabetes, start with a dose of 15 μg, which is 2½ units on an insulin syringe (0.3-cc syringe is recommended). If there are no clinically significant side effects, it is then safe to advance by 15 μg. If the patient experiences nausea or other GI side effects, do not increase the dose of pramlintide until the GI side effects dissipate. Patients with type 2 diabetes generally experience less GI side effects and their titration starts at 60 μg, followed by escalation to the final dose of 120 μg if the patient is asymptomatic.

■ Take Pramlintide Just Prior to the Meal

In a dose-timing study of pramlintide, postprandial glucose concentrations were lowered most effectively when pramlintide was administered just before the meal (**Figure 12.4**). This reduction of postprandial glucose occurred whether the patient was using insulin lispro or regular insulin.

■ When Initiating Pramlintide, Decrease Dose of Mealtime Insulin by 50%

Pramlintide not only works to reduce glucose appearance via the mechanisms previously described, but it may also lead to a reduction in food intake greater than anticipated by a patient newly starting pramlintide. Further adjustments of the insulin dose either up or down should be based on home glucose monitoring results and experience with pramlintide.

■ Timing of the Insulin Dose May Be Important

Many patients who have experience with pramlintide take a fast-acting insulin analog as they approach the end of a meal. The reason is because they will know how much and what types of food they have eaten, so the insulin dose calculation using carbohydrate counting or other means will be more accurate. Pramlintide delays gastric emptying and thus the peak in postprandial glucose may overlap with the peak action of the fast-acting analogs when given a little later than the beginning of the meal.

Future Trends

For patients with type 1 diabetes, pramlintide represents the first new agent to improve long-term glycemic control since the discovery of insulin nearly a century ago. Its addition to the therapeutic arsenal represents a potentially new era of diabetes management in which glucoregulatory hormones other than insulin will be used to more closely approximate normal glucohomeostasis in patients with diabetes. Several synthetic compounds with numerous capabilities for addressing the underlying pathophysiology of diabetes are being studied currently. The mechanisms of action of these agents include:

- Limiting the absorption of carbohydrates

- Enhancing the action of insulin at the level of target tissues
- Restricting glucose production by the liver
- Potentiating the secretory activity of the β-cell.

These new drugs, used in conjunction with analogues of insulin, amylin, or other glucoregulatory hormones, have great potential to improve the treatment of diabetes.

SUGGESTED READING

American College of Endocrinology. American College of Endocrinology Consensus Statement on Guidelines for Glycemic Control. *Endocr Pract*. 2002;8(suppl 1):5-11.

Brownlee M. Biochemistry and molecular cell biology of diabetic complications. *Nature*. 2001;414:813-820.

Buse JB, Weyer C, Maggs DG. Amylin replacement with Pramlintide in type 1 and type 2 diabetes: a physiological approach to overcome barriers with insulin therapy. *Clin Diabetes*. 2002;20:137-144.

Chapman I, Parker B, Doran S, et al. Effect of pramlintide on satiety and food intake in obese subjects and subjects with type 2 diabetes. *Diabetologia*. 2005;48:838-848.

Edelman SV, Weyer C. Unresolved challenges with insulin therapy in type 1 and type 2 diabetes: potential benefit of replacing amylin, a second beta-cell hormone. *Diabetes Technol Ther*. 2002;4:175-189.

Guthrie R, Karl D, Wang Y, et al. In an open-label clinical study pramlintide lowered A1C, body weight, and insulin use in patients with type 1 diabetes failing to achieve glycemic targets with insulin therapy. The 65th Annual Scientific Sessions of the American Diabetes Association; San Diego, Calfornia. June 10-14, 2005.

Heise T, Heinemann L, Heller S, et al. Effect of pramlintide on symptom, catecholamine, and glucagon responses to hypoglycemia in healthy subjects. *Metabolism*. 2004;53:1227-1232.

Hollander P, Maggs DG, Ruggles JA, et al. Effect of pramlintide on weight in overweight and obese insulin-treated type 2 diabetes patients. *Obes Res*. 2004;12:661-668.

Karl D, Wang Y, Lorenzi G, et al. In an open-label clinical study pramlintide lowered A1C, body weight, and insulin use in patients with type 2 diabetes failing to achieve glycemic targets with insulin therapy. The 65th Annual Scientific Sessions of the American Diabetes Association; San Diego, Calfornia. June 10-14, 2005.

Kolterman OG, Schwartz S, Corder C,et al. Effect of 14 days' subcutaneous administration of the human amylin analogue, pramlintide (AC137), on an intravenous insulin challenge and response to a standard liquid meal in patients with IDDM. *Diabetologia*. 1996;39:492-499.

Kruger DF, Gatcomb PM, Owen SK. Clinical implications of amylin and amylin deficiency. *Diabetes Educ*. 1999;25:389-397.

Maggs DG, Fineman M, Kornstein J, et al. Pramlintide reduces postprandial glucose excursions when added to insulin lispro in subjects with type 2 diabetes: a dose-timing study. *Diabetes Metab Res Rev*. 2004;20:55-60.

Nyholm B, Orskov L, Hove KY, et al. The amylin analog pramlintide improves glycemic control and reduces postprandial glucagon concentrations in patients with type 1 diabetes mellitus. *Metabolism*. 1999;48:935-941.

Saydah SH, Fradkin J, Cowie CC. Poor control of risk factors for vascular disease among adults with previously diagnosed diabetes. *JAMA*. 2004;291:335-342.

Scherbaum WA. The role of amylin in the physiology of glycemic control. *Exp Clin Endocrinol Diabetes*. 1998;106:97-102.

The relationship of glycemic exposure (HbA1c) to the risk of development and progression of retinopathy in the diabetes control and complications trial. *Diabetes*. 1995;44:968-983.

Weyer C, Gottlieb A, Kim DD, et al. Pramlintide reduces postprandial glucose excursions when added to regular insulin or insulin lispro in subjects with type 1 diabetes: a dose-timing study. *Diabetes Care*. 2003;26:3074-3079.

12

Whitehouse F, Kruger DF, Fineman M, et al. A randomized study and open-label extension evaluating the long-term efficacy of pramlintide as an adjunct to insulin therapy in type 1 diabetes. *Diabetes Care*. 2002;25:724-730.

Young AA, Gedulin BR, Rink TJ. Dose-responses for the slowing of gastric emptying in a rodent model by glucagon-like peptide (7-36) NH2, amylin, cholecystokinin, and other possible regulators of nutrient uptake. *Metabolism*. 1996;45:1-3.

13   Acute Complications

Patients with type 1 diabetes are prone to developing acute complications such as:

- Metabolic problems:
  - Diabetic ketoacidosis (DKA)
  - Hypoglycemia
- Infection
- Quality-of-life problems:
  - Nocturia
  - Poor sleep
  - Daytime tiredness
  - Tooth and gum disease
  - Cognitive impairment.

Common acute complications of type 1 diabetes are metabolic problems (DKA and hypoglycemia) and infection. In addition, the quality of life of patients with frequent severe hypoglycemia is adversely affected. Characteristic symptoms of tiredness and lethargy can be significant and lead to increased falls and bedsores in the elderly, urinary tract infections, decreased school performance in children, and decreased work performance in adults.

Diabetic Ketoacidosis

Diabetic ketoacidosis is an acute life-threatening complication of diabetes resulting from profound insulin deficiency, such as that seen in uncontrolled and newly diagnosed type 1 diabetes. The annual incidence of DKA in the United States is estimated at five to eight episodes per 1,000 people with diabetes. Two percent to 8% of all diabetes-related hospital admissions are attributed to DKA, but with the availability of self-monitoring of blood glucose (SMBG), DKA is apt to be recognized in the early stages when sufficient urgent treatment may be administered in an office or clinic setting. Nevertheless, mortality rates for DKA have remained within the range of 2% to 10% over the past 30 years. In patients >65 years of age, the mortality rate for DKA exceeds 20%, a statistic worth noting given that the number of people diagnosed with type 1 diabetes later in life is increasing.

Key characteristics of DKA include:

- Hyperglycemia (300 to 800 mg/dL, although usually <600 mg/dL. The glucose concentration is not related to severity of DKA.)
- Ketosis: serum ketones usually 10 to 20 mM and acidosis (pH 6.8-7.3, HCO_3 <15 mEq/L)
- Dehydration caused by:
  - Nausea
  - Vomiting
  - Inadequate oral intake
  - Electrolyte depletion (eg, potassium, magnesium, etc).

Precipitating factors of DKA are listed in **Table 13.1**. They vary from patient to patient and may include the following (approximately 50% of which are preventable):

- Illness and infection; increased production of glucagons and glucocorticoids by adrenal gland promotes gluconeogenesis; increased production of epinephrine and norepinephrine increases glycogenolysis
- Inadequate insulin dosage due to omission or reduction of doses by patient, physician, or clinic; patients with gastrointestinal (GI) distress often decrease or eliminate their insulin doses thinking that less insulin is needed when food intake is decreased; this practice can be dangerous because GI symptoms are key features of DKA

TABLE 13.1 — Triggers for Hyperglycemia, Ketosis, and Diabetic Ketoacidosis

- New-onset diabetes
- Infection
- Trauma
- Surgery
- Emotional stress
- Errors in insulin administration
- Pump failure
- Intentional manipulation of insulin dosing
- Myocardial infarction
- Medications
- Substance abuse
- Eating disorders
- Comorbidities

Laffel L. *Endocrinol Metab Clin North Am.* 2000;29:709.

- Initial manifestation of type 1 diabetes
- Chronic untreated hyperglycemia (glucose toxicity) and hyperinsulinemia

■ Pathophysiology of DKA

Diabetic ketoacidosis is a metabolic acidosis caused by significant insulin deficiency. The following physiologic abnormalities are characteristic of DKA and require prompt correction:

- Chronic hyperglycemia and glucose toxicity
- Acidosis caused by catabolism of fat and the buildup of ketone bodies
- Low blood volume because of dehydration (loss of fluid and electrolytes)
- Hyperosmolality because of renal water loss and water depletion from sweating, nausea, and vomiting, and associated potassium loss.

■ Symptoms and Signs of DKA

The classic symptoms and signs of DKA in type 1 diabetes are shown in **Table 13.2**. Polyuria and poly-

TABLE 13.2 — Symptoms and Signs of Classic Diabetic Ketoacidosis

Symptoms of DKA
- Nausea
- Vomiting
- Abdominal pain
- Dyspnea
- Myalgia
- Headache
- Anorexia
- Characteristic symptoms of hyperglycemia
- Hypothermia

Signs of DKA
- Hypothermia
- Hyperpnea (Kussmaul's respiration)
- Acetone breath
- Dehydration (intravascular volume depletion hypotension)
- Hyporeflexia
- Acute abdomen (tenderness to palpation, muscle guarding, diminished bowel sounds)
- Stupor (mild to frank coma)
- Hypotonia
- Uncoordinated ocular movements

Abbreviation: DKA, diabetic ketoacidosis.

Davidson MB. *Diabetes Mellitus: Diagnosis and Treatment*, 3rd ed. New York, NY: Churchill Livingstone; 1991:192.

dipsia are symptoms of osmotic diuresis secondary to hyperglycemia. Nonspecific symptoms include weakness, lethargy, headache, and myalgia; specific symptoms of DKA are GI and respiratory. The GI symptoms probably are related to the ketosis and/or acidosis. The chief respiratory complaint of dyspnea actually is an inability to catch one's breath. This type of hyperventilation unrelated to exertion is the ventilatory response to metabolic acidosis termed Kussmaul's respiration. Ketone bodies cause the breath to smell fruity.

Because the signs are not specific to DKA, physicians should be alert to a constellation of evidence that points to the possibility of DKA.

Because other diseases and conditions may mimic DKA and precipitate and/or coexist with DKA, the following differential diagnoses (and representative DKA symptoms) should be considered:

- Cerebrovascular accident (altered mental status)
- Brainstem hemorrhage (hyperventilation, glucosuria)
- Hypoglycemia (altered mental status, tachycardia)
- Metabolic acidosis (hyperventilation, anion-gap acidosis):
  - Uremia
  - Salicylate
  - Methanol
  - Ethylene glycol
- Gastroenteritis (nausea, vomiting, abdominal pain)
- Acute abdomen
- Pneumonia (hyperventilation).

■ Laboratory Evaluation

A definitive diagnosis of DKA is based on the following evaluations: plasma glucose, blood urea nitrogen/creatinine, serum ketones, electrolytes (with calculated anion gap), osmolality, urinalysis, urine ketones by dipstick, as well as initial arterial blood gases, complete blood count with differential, and electrocardiogram. Bacterial cultures of urine, blood, and throat, etc, should be performed to determine the presence of infection. A chest x-ray should also be obtained. **Table 13.3** shows typical laboratory findings in patients with DKA.

Most patients in hyperglycemic crisis present with leukocytosis proportional to blood ketone body concentration. Serum sodium concentration is usually decreased because of the osmotic flux of water from the

TABLE 13.3 — Diagnostic Criteria for Diabetic Ketoacidosis

	Diabetic Ketoacidosis		
	Mild	Moderate	Severe
Plasma glucose (mg/dL)	>250	>250	>250
Arterial pH	7.25 to 7.30	7.00 to 7.24	<7.00
Serum bicarbonate (mEq/L)	15 to 18	10 to <15	<10
Urine ketones*	Positive	Positive	Positive
Serum ketones*	Positive	Positive	Positive
Effective serum osmolality (mOsm/kg)[†]	Variable	Variable	Variable
Anion gap[‡]	>10	>12	>12
Alteration in sensorial or obtundation	Alert	Alert/drowsy	Stupor/coma

* Nitroprusside reaction method.

† Calculation: $2 \times$ measured Na (mEq/L) + glucose (mg/dL)/18.

‡ Calculation: $(Na^+) - (Cl^- + HCO_3^-)$ (mEq/L).

Adapted from: *Diabetes Care.* 2003;26:S109-S117.

intracellular to the extracellular space when hyperglycemia is present. Occasionally, serum sodium concentration may be falsely lowered by severe hypertriglyceridemia. Serum potassium concentration may be elevated because of an extracellular shift of potassium resulting from insulin deficiency, hypertonicity, and acidemia. Patients with low-normal or low serum potassium concentration on admission have severe total-body potassium deficiency and require very careful monitoring and more aggressive potassium replacement, because treatment lowers potassium further and can lead to cardiac dysrhythmia. The occurrence of stupor or coma in the absence of definitive elevation of effective osmolality (>320 mOsm/kg) warrants immediate consideration of other possible causes of mental status change. Effective osmolality may be calculated by the following formula:

$$2 \times \text{measured Na (mEq/L)} + \text{glucose (mg/dL)}/18$$

Amylase levels are elevated in the majority of patients with DKA, but this may be due to causes involving organs other than the pancreas (eg, the parotid gland). A serum lipase determination may be beneficial in the differential diagnosis of pancreatitis.

13

Differential Diagnosis

Patients may have ketoacidosis without DKA. Starvation ketosis and alcoholic ketoacidosis (AKA) are differentiated by clinical history and by plasma glucose concentrations that range from mildly elevated (rare >250 mg/dL) to hypoglycemia. While AKA can lead to serious acidosis, the serum bicarbonate concentration in starvation ketosis usually does not fall below 18 mEq/L. DKA must also be distinguished from other causes of high anion-gap metabolic acidosis (eg, ingestion of substances such as salicylate, methanol, ethylene glycol, and paraldehyde), chronic renal failure, and lactic acidosis. Clinical history of previous drug intoxications or metformin use should be obtained. Measurement of blood lactate, serum salicylate, and blood methanol level can be useful.

■ Treatment

Treatment of diabetic ketoacidosis centers on hydration, insulin use, electrolyte replenishment, and prevention of future episodes (sick-day management). Precipitating causes should be identified and treated concurrently. Successive changes in the patient's condition must be documented in a flow sheet (**Table 13.4**).

Fluid Therapy

The type of fluids and rate at which they should be infused are issues of ongoing debate in the treatment of hyperglycemic crisis. Initially, these should be determined by the volume status of the patient. Supine hypotension indicates an approximate decrease of 20% in extracellular fluid, while orthostatic hypotension signifies a 15% to 20% reduction in extracellular volume. An orthostatic elevation in pulse unaccompanied by a change in blood pressure suggests a 10% decrease. In all of these cases, there is consensus that the first fluid infused should be 0.0% normal saline administered as quickly as possible over the first hour, followed by 500 to 1000 mL/hour for the next 2 hours of either 0.9% normal saline or 0.45% normal saline, depending on the hydration and serum sodium levels. Although one school of thought advocates hypotonic saline (0.45% normal saline) from the outset if the effective serum osmolality (calculated by $2 \times$ measured sodium [mEq/L] + glucose [mg/dL]/18) is >320, we prefer the initial use of 0.9% saline for the first hour followed by 0.45% saline, unless volume losses are severe and hypotension is not corrected after the first liter of fluid.

TABLE 13.4 — Ketoacidosis Flow Sheet	
	Monitoring Interval (hours)
Clinical	
Mental status	1
Vital signs (T, P, R, BP)	1
ECG	Initially and as indicated
Weight	Initially and daily
Therapy	
Fluid intake and output (mL/h)	4
Insulin (U/h)	1
Potassium (mEq/h)	4
Glucose (g/h)	4
Bicarbonate and phosphate (mEq/h)	4
Laboratory	
Glucose (bedside)	1
Potassium, pH	2
Sodium, chloride, bicarbonate	4
Phosphate, magnesium	4
BUN or creatinine	4

Abbreviations: BP, blood pressure; BUN, blood urea nitrogen; ECG, electrocardiogram; P, pulse; R, respirations; T, temperature.

Bode BW, ed. *Medical Management of Type 1 Diabetes*. 4th ed. New York, NY: McGraw-Hill; 2004:129.

13

Dextrose (5%) should be added to the solution when blood glucose reaches 250 mg/dL in DKA for two primary reasons. First, it allows continued insulin administration to control ketogenesis in DKA. Second, especially in pediatric patients, too rapid a decrease in blood glucose can cause cerebral edema. Additionally, once blood pressure is stabilized and glucose levels decrease to the point that osmotic diuresis is not causing further water and electrolyte losses, urine volume will also diminish, allowing a tapering of intravenous (IV) fluids. This is critical in young children and the elderly, both of whom are at greater risk for overhydration and attendant cerebral edema. The precise fluid rate must be determined on a case-by-case basis, but usually ranges from 4 to 14 mL/kg/hour. The average length of time necessary for IV hydration is about 48 hours, but this varies greatly from patient to patient.

Insulin Infusion

Before starting insulin therapy for DKA, it is important to confirm the level of electrolytes. In the relatively unusual circumstance of hypokalemia, insulin therapy must be postponed until potassium levels are corrected. Although approaches vary, insulin infusion (all human regular insulin) normally begins with an IV bolus of 0.1 to 0.15 U/kg, followed by 0.1 U/kg/hour. Some endocrinologists prefer intramuscular insulin at 7 to 10 U except when hypotension is present, in which case only IV administration will ensure adequate absorption. Sometimes insulin resistance will require much larger doses of insulin than those specified here, but even low doses of insulin will inhibit lipolysis and ketogenesis. The insulin infusion rate can be decreased when blood glucose measures 250 to 300 mg/dL, at which time dextrose (5%) may be added, as previously described. Blood glucose should be measured hourly, while electrolytes may be evaluated less frequently. If blood glucose levels fail to drop 50 to 70 mg/dL/hour, it is necessary to investigate possible causes, such as an error in the insulin infusion mixture.

Potassium

Patients with DKA are depleted in total-body potassium, although their serum potassium level may be normal or even elevated. Often, patients presenting with DKA have a potassium deficit of 500 to 700 mEq/L, which must be replaced to a minimum level of 3.3 mEq/L before initiation of insulin therapy. This is because IV insulin moves potassium from extracellular to intracellular domains, while IV fluids increase renal plasma flow. Patients presenting with hypokalemia should be monitored with telemetry. In general, potassium replacement should not exceed 40 mEq the first hour and then 20 to 30 mEq per each subsequent hour.

Bicarbonate

The addition of bicarbonate remains a topic of debate in the treatment of DKA. Often, acidemia will improve as bicarbonate is produced by the liver in response to insulin therapy and reversal of ketogenesis. Some authorities maintain that because the addition of bicarbonate will result in more severe altered consciousness and headache in children and, certainly, more serious hypokalemia, its use should be limited to treatment of life-threatening hyperkalemia. However, controlled trials examining use of bicarbonate therapy for severe acidemia have led the American Diabetes Association to recommend it for patients who present with a pH <7.0. The solution should be infused as 1 ampule (50 mmol) with another solution, such as 0.45% normal saline. It should never be given as a bolus.

Phosphate

As with potassium, initial levels of serum phosphate are often normal or increased, even when there is a total-body deficit. Insulin therapy causes a migration of phosphate into the cell, causing hypophosphatemia during treatment. However, this rarely poses a problem unless serum phosphate falls below 1 mg/dL. Furthermore, controlled trials have not demonstrated a benefit from routine use of phosphate therapy for DKA. Current guidelines call for replacing phosphate if levels decrease below 1.0 mg/dL by adding 20 to 30 mEq/L of potassium phosphate to the IV solution over 2 to 3 hours. Serum calcium levels should be checked to avoid hypocalcemia, which is a potential complication.

Treatment Complications

Treatment complications include cerebral edema, hypoxemia, and noncardiogenic pulmonary edema. Cerebral edema occurs in 0.7% to 1.0% of children with DKA. Neurologic deterioration can be rapid, with headache, lethargy, and progressive decrease in arousal, leading to seizures, bradycardia, and respiratory arrest. Once symptoms progress beyond lethargy, a mortality risk of >70% has been shown and permanent morbidity is estimated at 86% to 93%.

Reduction in colloid osmotic pressure leading to increased pulmonary water content and decreased lung compliance is associated with hypoxemia. Patients with rales on exam are at higher risk for developing pulmonary edema.

■ Prevention of Diabetic Ketoacidosis (Sick-Day Management)

To prevent future DKA episodes, patients should be aware of "sick-day rules." The key components of sick-day management are:

- Continuation of insulin therapy
- Frequent monitoring of blood glucose
- Monitoring for ketosis
- Providing supplemental fast-acting or rapid-acting insulin doses according to home glucose monitoring algorithms
- Treating the underlying disorder
- Frequent contact with the medical team to review clinical status.

Continuation of Insulin Therapy

Illness poses a number of issues for patients with type 1 diabetes and their families. Insulin must always be given during illness, despite marked decreases in food intake. Infection induces insulin resistance, often necessitating increased or supplemental doses of insulin. In general, the patient should receive the normally prescribed dose supplemented by regular or rapid-acting insulin. Rapid-acting insulins are greatly preferred because of their faster onset of action. Supplemental insulin doses, generally 10% to 20% of the total daily insulin dose, are based on blood glucose level and urine ketone results (**Table 13.5**). Supplements of regular insulin may need to be administered every 3 to 4 hours; supplements of lispro or aspart may need to be repeated at 2- to 3-hour intervals. Frequent monitoring is essential and reductions in the insulin dose may be needed as the patient's illness improves. The key to successful treatment is vigilant blood glucose testing and administration of frequent small doses of a fast-acting insulin analogue to keep glycemia <200 mg/dL. If prolonged illness is expected, adjustment of basal insulin upward by 10% to 20% may be needed.

Prevention of Dehydration and Hypoglycemia

13

Fluid intake is necessary to prevent dehydration. Oral hydration is preferred but may be impossible if nausea and vomiting are present. If vomiting occurs, the health care team should be contacted immediately. Attempts at oral hydration with frequent small quantities of clear fluids are advised. The use of antiemetics may also be warranted. When anorexia is present and solid food intake is reduced or absent, sugar-containing drinks (eg, regular soda, clear juices, or flavored sugar-containing gelatin) are recommended, especially when blood glucose is <180 to 200 mg/dL. Volumes

TABLE 13.5 — Supplemental Insulin Doses Based on Blood Glucose and Urine Ketone Results

| Urine Ketones | Blood Glucose Level (mg/dL) | | | |
(more than a trace)	<80	80-250	250-400	>400
No	Omit regular or lispro/aspart when po intake is decreased	Usual dose	10% of TDD	20% of TDD
Yes	Decrease intermediate insulin by 20%; contact health care team, especially if vomiting occurs	Usual dose	20% of TDD	20% of TDD

Note: Suggested supplemental insulin may be given as regular or lispro. Total daily dose (TDD) is calculated by adding up all of the insulin administered on a usual day, including the fast- or rapid-acting insulin and the intermediate or long-acting insulin. Do not include supplements added to the usual dose because of unexpected hyperglycemia.

Adapted from: Laffel L. *Endocrinol Metab Clin North Am.* 2000;29:715.

of 3 to 8 oz/hour or, for children, 2 mL/lb of body weight per hour or $3 L/m^2/day$ should be encouraged. Even if the glucose values are high, extra doses of rapid-acting lispro or aspart may be administered to compensate for the glucose-containing nutrients. When GI losses from vomiting or diarrhea occur, liquids containing salt and potassium are recommended.

Sugar-free drinks are advised when the patient can take in solids that supply adequate carbohydrates and calories. Additionally, antipyretics are needed if fever is present to reduce further fluid loss. In addition to keeping oral antipyretics on hand, suppositories containing antiemetics should be available during periods of nausea and vomiting.

An evaluation of hydration status is important to avoid decompensation. Signs and symptoms of dehydration should be monitored and treated promptly and aggressively.

Monitor Blood Glucose Frequently

Self-monitoring, or monitoring of blood glucose by a family member or significant other, is necessary at least every 2 to 4 hours and should be done more frequently if blood glucose levels are low. Keeping careful records to trace illness progression and detect early signs of decompensation can prevent onset or recurrence of frank ketoacidosis.

Monitor for Ketosis

Urine tests for ketones are an important component of monitoring for sick-day management. This should be done at 3- to 4-hour intervals during illness, with stress, or whenever blood glucose levels are consistently >300 mg/dL. (Meters for home-monitoring of blood ketones, such as the Precision Xtra [Medisense, Bedford, Mass], are now available.) Appropriate storage of supplies and the use of insulin algorithms based on blood glucose and urine ketone results are essential. Supplemental insulin administration and hydration are generally adequate to treat ketosis successfully. If urine ketones are not cleared within 12 hours, a health care professional should be contacted.

Provide Supplemental Fast-Acting or Rapid-Acting Insulin

In general, the presence of ketones is a signal of insulin deficiency and the need for supplemental insulin. In the setting of GI illness associated with vomiting, diarrhea, increased transit time, and malabsorption, there is always the potential for hypoglycemia; however, hyperglycemia is the rule rather than the exception. If hypoglycemia is an issue, especially when blood glucose values are <80 mg/dL in the setting of positive ketones, it is necessary to increase fluid and carbohydrate intake (10 to 15 g) until blood glucose increases. Fluid intake should be maintained until the ketones clear.

Supplemental doses of fast-acting (regular) or, preferably, rapid-acting (lispro or aspart) insulin should be administered whenever hyperglycemia and ketosis are present. The degree of hyperglycemia and the presence or absence of urinary ketones indicate the doses and frequency of supplemental insulin. The doses are generally calculated according to the patient's weight, ranging from 0.1 to 0.3 U/kg, usually between 10% and 20% of the total daily insulin requirement in the baseline state, or according to a team-derived algorithm (**Table 13.6**). An algorithms for patients treated with continuous subcutaneous insulin infusion is shown in **Table 13.7**. The health care team should individualize the approach according to the patient's insulin sensitivity, the severity and duration of the illness, and the presence of anorexia. If blood glucose remains elevated, with or without positive urine ketones, addi-

TABLE 13.6 — Alternative Algorithm for Supplemental Regular or Rapid-Acting Insulin Doses Incorporating More Complexity

Urine Ketones	Blood Glucose Level (mg/dL)*		
	<250	250-400	>400
Negative/trace	No change	5%	10%
Small	0% to 5%	10%	15%
Moderate/large	0% to 10%	15% to 20%	20%

* If blood glucose level is <80 mg/dL and po intake is decreased, omit regular or rapid-acting insulin and decrease intermediate-acting insulin by 20%. Contact health care team, especially if vomiting occurs.

Adapted from: Laffel L. *Endocrinol Metab Clin North Am.* 2000;29:718.

13

TABLE 13.7 — Continuous Subcutaneous Insulin Infusion Sick-Day Management

- Never omit basal insulin. Do not disconnect or stop insulin pump unless patient is receiving insulin by injection.
- Increase frequency of blood glucose and urine ketone monitoring to every 2 to 4 hours throughout the entire day and night.
- During illness, increase basal rate by 20% to 50% until illness resolves and blood glucose levels are back in range.
- Adjust boluses to carbohydrate intake. Increase premeal boluses by 20% to 50% as needed to return blood glucose levels to their target range.
- Increase fluid intake as needed to help clear ketones.
- Examine infusion site as possible source of occult infection and cause of hyperglycemia and ketosis.
- Check pump and infusion device. If blood glucose levels and ketones remain elevated for >3 to 4 hours, give supplemental insulin by syringe or pen. Determine dose according to "correction factor" or as 20% of usual total daily insulin dose. Change pump infusion set-up.
- Call health care team if patient has persistent nausea or vomiting for >4 hours, if symptoms of diabetic ketoacidosis develop (chest or abdominal pain, deep breathing), or if questions or concerns arise.

Laffel L. *Endocrinol Metab Clin North Am.* 2000;29:719.

tional supplemental insulin doses may be needed every 3 to 4 hours. If rapid-acting insulin is administered, doses may need to be repeated at 2 to 3 hourly intervals. Patients (or their family members) should continue to monitor and record blood glucose and ketones every 2 to 4 hours.

Treat Underlying Triggers

Any acute infection should be evaluated and treated accordingly. Intercurrent viral illnesses for which there is no prescriptive treatment may still require sick-day management. Symptomatic treatment with antipyretics and analgesics is helpful. Patients with a history of recurrent DKA, known eating disorders, psychosocial problems, or poorly controlled blood glucose are at risk for decompensation and should be encouraged to contact their health care team when signs and symptoms of illness first appear. If access to a telephone or transportation is difficult, appropriate arrangements should be made in advance.

Frequent Contact With Health Care Team

Patients and their family members should be on the alert for signs and symptoms indicating that medical attention is required. These include:

- Continued vomiting >2 to 4 hours in duration
- Blood glucose persistently exceeding 300 mg/dL and unable to be lowered with frequent doses of insulin or persistent ketones for >12 hours
- Signs of dehydration such as:
  - Dry mouth
  - Cracked lips
  - Weight loss
  - Sunken eyes
  - Dry skin
- Symptoms suggesting development of DKA, such as:
  - Nausea
  - Abdominal or chest pain
  - Vomiting
  - Ketotic breath
  - Hyperventilation
  - Altered consciousness.

The latter symptoms, in particular, warrant emergency medical attention. If identified early, milder forms of DKA can be treated in the outpatient setting.

Hypoglycemia

This metabolic problem occurs when there is an imbalance between food intake and the appropriate dosage and timing of insulin therapy. Other factors that contribute to hypoglycemia are:

- Exercise (planned or unplanned)
- Undernutrition or delayed meals
- Inappropriate dose of insulin
- Inappropriate timing of insulin dose
- Erratic absorption of insulin
- Surreptitious administration of insulin
- Excessive alcohol intake on an empty stomach
- Other drugs and medication
- Decreased liver or kidney function.

■ Signs of Hypoglycemia

Hypoglycemia should be suspected in patients who demonstrate the following clinical signs; a diagnosis of hypoglycemia is confirmed in a symptomatic patient if a plasma glucose level <60 mg/dL occurs:

- Mild hypoglycemia is associated with adrenergic or cholinergic symptoms such as:
  - Pallor
  - Diaphoresis
  - Tachycardia
  - Palpitations
  - Hunger
  - Paresthesias
  - Shakiness
- Moderate hypoglycemia (<40 mg/dL) is associated with neuroglycopenic symptoms of altered mental and/or neurologic functioning such as:
  - Inability to concentrate
  - Confusion
  - Slurred speech
  - Irrational or uncontrolled behavior
  - Slowed reaction time

- Blurred vision
- Somnolence
- Extreme fatigue

• Severe hypoglycemia (<20 mg/dL) is associated with extreme impairment of neurologic function to the extent that the assistance of another person is needed to obtain treatment; symptoms include:
  - Completely automatic/disoriented behavior
  - Loss of consciousness
  - Inability to arouse from sleep
  - Seizures
  - Death.

It is important to understand that hypoglycemia does not necessarily progress in a linear fashion from mild to severe. For example, some patients might develop neuroglycopenic symptoms before adrenergic or cholinergic symptoms, and other patients may overlook or ignore adrenergic or cholinergic symptoms and progress to neuroglycopenia. In many patients, hypoglycemia unawareness becomes a significant problem as the result of defective counterregulatory responses associated with reduced or absent glucagon secretion. This defect, which can emerge 3 to 5 years from diagnosis, is considered an important clinical problem because current diabetes management with intensive insulin regimens usually increases the risk and frequency of hypoglycemic events.

13

■ **Treatment**

The goal of treatment is to normalize the plasma glucose level as quickly as possible.

• Mild hypoglycemia is treated most effectively by having the patient ingest approximately 15 g of readily available carbohydrate by mouth. Sources of carbohydrate (15 g) include:
  - Three glucose tablets (5 g each)

- $^1/_2$ cup fruit juice
- 2 tablespoons raisins
- 5 Lifesavers® candies
- $^1/_2$ to $^3/_4$ cup regular soda (not diet)
- 1 cup milk

If symptoms continue, treatment may need to be repeated in 15 minutes. Most patients can resume normal activity following treatment.

- For moderate hypoglycemia, larger amounts of carbohydrate (15 to 30 g) that are rapidly absorbed may be needed. Patients usually are instructed to consume additional food after the initial treatment and wait approximately 30 minutes until resuming activity. Measuring blood glucose levels during treatment and the recovery period can help determine the effectiveness of treatment. Some patients, however, may continue to have neuroglycopenic symptoms for an hour or longer after blood glucose levels have increased >100 mg/dL.

- Severe hypoglycemia, where patients are completely incapacitated, requires rapid treatment. IV glucose (50 cc 50% dextrose or glucose followed by 10% dextrose drip) is the most effective routine; however, glucagon (1 mg for adults) can be administered intramuscularly at home with positive results. Individuals who are unable to swallow should be given glucagon or glucose gel, honey, syrup, or jelly on the inside of the cheek. After the initial response, a rapid-acting, carbohydrate-containing liquid should be given until nausea subsides; then a small snack or meal can be consumed. Blood glucose levels should be monitored frequently for several hours to assure that the levels remain normal and to avoid overtreatment. The individual's health care team should be informed of any severe hypoglycemic episodes.

- It is important to educate patients on the proper treatment of hypoglycemia. For example, many eat candy bars that contain excessive amounts of fat and calories, thus leading to delayed recovery from hypoglycemia and unnecessary weight gain.

■ Prevention of Hypoglycemia

Patients can take certain measures to avoid hypoglycemia:

- Know the signs and symptoms of hypoglycemia.
- Try to eat meals on a regular schedule.
- Try to eat the same amounts and types of food as much as possible.
- Carry a source of carbohydrate (at least 10 to 15 g)
- Perform SMBG regularly for early detection of low blood glucose levels; initiate treatment at the first signs of hypoglycemia. Patients should be made aware of when hypoglycemic reactions are most likely to occur (ie, when the insulin(s) is peaking).
- Take regular insulin at least 30 minutes before eating. (Patients who take their regular insulin immediately before or after the meal will be prone to delayed hypoglycemia.) A fast-acting insulin analogue should be taken 5 minutes before consumption of the meal.
- Schedule exercise appropriately; adjust meal times, calorie intake, or insulin dosing to accommodate physical activity; use SMBG (before, during, after strenuous activity) to determine the effect of exercise on blood glucose levels and to detect low blood glucose levels.
- Check blood glucose level before going to sleep to avoid nocturnal hypoglycemia; perform nocturnal (3 AM) monitoring:
  – If hypoglycemia has occurred during the night

13

217

- When evening insulin has been adjusted
- When strenuous activity has occurred the previous day
- During times of irregular eating schedules or erratic glucose control
- Several nutrition bars that are low in fat have been developed to help prevent hypoglycemia (Extend Bar).

SUGGESTED READING

Bode BW, ed. *Medical Management of Type 1 Diabetes*. 4th ed. New York, NY: McGraw-Hill; 2004.

Kitabchi AE, Umpierrez GE, Murphy MB, et al. Hyperglycemic crisis in patients with diabetes mellitus. *Diabetes Care*. 2003;26(suppl 1):S109-S117.

Laffel L. Sick-day management in type 1 diabetes. *Endocrinol Metab Clin North Am*. 2000;29:707-723.

Peragallo-Dittko V, ed. *A Core Curriculum for Diabetes Education*. 2nd ed. Chicago, Ill: American Association of Diabetes Educators; 1993.

Porte D, Sherwin RS. *Ellenberg and Rifkin's Diabetes Mellitus*. 5th ed. Stamford, Conn: Appleton and Lange; 1997.

14 Long-Term Complications

The long-term complications that may develop in patients with type 1 diabetes include:

- Microvascular disease
  - Diabetic retinopathy
  - Diabetic nephropathy
  - Diabetic neuropathy
    - Symmetric distal neuropathy
    - Mononeuropathy
    - Diabetic amyotrophy
    - Gastroparesis
    - Diabetic diarrhea
    - Neurogenic bladder
    - Impaired cardiovascular (CV) reflexes (sudden death)
    - Sexual dysfunction
- Macrovascular disease
  - Hypertension
  - Dyslipidemia
- Diabetic foot disorders.

The long-term, chronic complications of diabetes have the greatest impact on the health of individuals with diabetes as well as on the health care system. Diabetes and its associated vascular complications are the fourth leading cause of death in the United States. Consequently, early detection and aggressive treatment of these complications are essential to reduce associated morbidity and mortality. Striving for tight metabolic control also has been proven to help delay the onset and prevent the development of microvascular complications (diabetic retinopathy, nephropathy, and neuropathy).

14

The Diabetes Control and Complications Trial (DCCT), a multicenter, randomized clinical trial, investigated the effects of intensive therapy vs traditional therapy on the development and progression of microvascular complications of type 1 diabetes mellitus. The aim of intensive therapy was to achieve and maintain near-normal blood glucose values following a regimen of three or more daily insulin injections or treatment with an insulin pump. In contrast, only one or two insulin injections were used in conventional therapy. Patients were followed for a mean of 6.5 years and assessed regularly for the presence or progression of retinopathy, nephropathy, and neuropathy.

Intensive therapy proved to be highly effective in delaying the onset and slowing the progression of the long-term complications being evaluated in patients with type 1 diabetes. Furthermore, similar benefits were observed in the United Kingdom Prospective Diabetes Study (UKPDS) in type 2 diabetes. In response to the DCCT and UKPDS findings, the American Diabetes Association (ADA) recommended striving for the best possible glycemic control in patients with type 1 and type 2 diabetes, with the following goals:

- Fasting and preprandial blood glucose level of 90 mg/dL to 130 mg/dL
- Postprandial glucose level of <180 mg/dL
- Glycosylated hemoglobin (A1C) of <7% (normal reference range = 4% to 6%) or three standard deviations from the mean of the normal range.

Attempts to normalize glycemia and glycosylated hemoglobin should be balanced, however, with minimizing weight gain and hypoglycemia, and maintaining an acceptable quality of life.

Although the mechanisms of microvascular complications are multifactorial, chronic hyperglycemia is a prerequisite (**Figure 14.1**). Excess glucose combines with free amino acids on serum or tissue proteins, eventually forming irreversible advanced glycosylation product (AGE) in diabetic patients. Elevated circulating AGE concentrations increase vascular permeability, promote the influx of mononuclear cells, stimulate cell proliferation, and, apparently, modify low-density lipoprotein (LDL). Additionally, glucose metabolism via the enzyme aldose reductase is amplified with chronic hyperglycemia, causing sorbitol to accumulate within cells. The result is a rise in intracellular osmolality and a decrease in intracellular myoinositol, both of which can disrupt cell metabolism. Another possible contributing factor is activation of isomers of protein kinase C (PKC) by more pronounced synthesis of diacylglycerol. Thus PKC inhibitors are now being tested for treatment of a number of vascular complications.

Retinopathy, nephropathy, and neuropathy are the major microvascular complications of diabetes. Prevention, early detection, and aggressive treatment are essential to reduce associated morbidity and mortality. Stringent glycemic control has been clearly shown to prevent the development or delay the progression of these complications in both types of diabetes.

14

■ Diabetic Retinopathy
The development and progression of retinopathy depends on the duration of diabetes and the duration and severity of hyperglycemia. Because diabetic retinopathy does not cause symptoms until it has reached an advanced stage, early and frequent evaluation for vision problems is critical for patients with diabetes.

FIGURE 14.1 — Possible Molecular Mechanisms of Diabetes-Related Complications

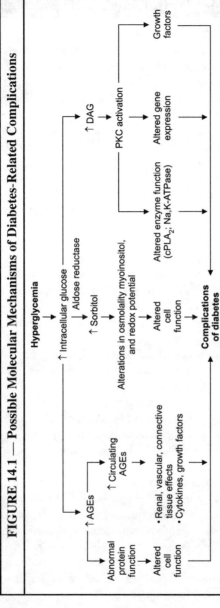

Abbreviations: AGE, advanced glycation end product; cPLA$_2$, phospholipase A$_2$; DAG, diacylglycerol; NA,K-ATPase, sodium-potassium ATPase; PKC, protein kinase C.

Braunwald E, et al, eds. *Harrison's Principles of Internal Medicine.* 15th ed. New York, NY: The McGraw-Hill Companies; 2001:2120.

The following findings also support the importance of early detection:

- Diabetes is the leading cause of all new cases of blindness (13%)
- Loss of vision associated with diabetic retinopathy and macular edema can be reduced by at least 50% with laser photocoagulation if identified in a timely manner.

Nonproliferative

Background changes are the earliest stage of retinopathy and are characterized by microaneurysms and intraretinal "dot and blot" hemorrhages (**Figure 14**.2). If serous fluid leaks into the area of the maculae (where central vision originates), macular edema can occur and cause disruption in light transmission and visual acuity. Macular edema cannot be observed directly but is suggested by the presence of hard exudates close to the maculae. Any of these findings should prompt immediate referral to an ophthalmologist.

Preproliferative

Advanced background retinopathy with certain lesions is considered the preproliferative stage and indicates an increased risk of progression to proliferative retinopathy. This stage is characterized by:

- "Beading" of the retinal veins
- Soft exudates (also called "cotton-wool" spots that are ischemic infarcts of the inner retinal layers) (**Figure 14**.3)
- Irregular, dilated, tortuous retinal capillaries or occasionally newly formed intraretinal vessels.

Any of these signs suggests the need for further evaluation by an ophthalmologist.

14

**FIGURE 14.2 — Background
Diabetic Retinopathy**

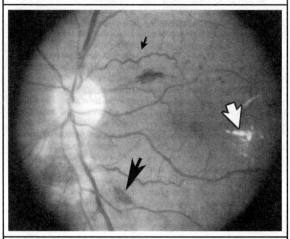

Note microaneurysm *(small black arrow)*, hard exudate *(white arrow)*, and hemorrhage *(large black arrow)*.

Courtesy of Albert Sheffer, MD.

Proliferative

Proliferative retinopathy is the final stage of this degenerative condition and imparts the most serious threat to vision. Neovascularization typically covers more than one third of the optic disk and may extend into the posterior vitreous. These fragile new vessels, which are prone to bleeding, probably develop in response to ischemia. Bleeding that occurs in the vitreous or preretinal space can cause visual symptoms, such as "floaters" or "cobwebs," or retinal detachment that results from contraction of fibrous tissue. Sudden and painless vision loss usually is related to a major retinal hemorrhage.

FIGURE 14.3 — Preproliferative Retinopathy

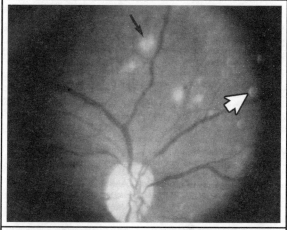

The soft or cotton-wool exudate *(black arrow)* has indistinct margins in contrast to the hard exudate in Figure 14.2, which has sharp margins and is brighter. The round structures with distinct margins *(white arrow)* are artifacts.

Courtesy of Albert Sheffer, MD.

Evaluation and Referral

Because visual acuity frequently changes in response to fluctuations in glycemic control (particularly extreme variations, eg, low-to-high and high-to-low), the reason for any vision changes should be thoroughly investigated. All patients with diabetes should have annual eye examinations with complete visual history, visual acuity examinations, and careful ophthalmoscopic examinations with a dilated pupil. Patients with type 1 diabetes should begin having annual eye examinations after 5 years of diabetes postpuberty.

Treatment

Treatment of nonproliferative and preproliferative retinopathy typically involves blood glucose control and blood pressure control. The only standard treatment for background retinopathy, in addition to optimizing metabolic control and blood pressure, is photocoagulation treatment. Results of the Early Treatment Diabetic Retinopathy Study revealed the effectiveness of argon laser photocoagulation applied focally (eg, spot-welding the leaking microaneurysms) in treating macular edema and stabilizing vision. Photocoagulation can slow the progression of vision loss in cases of macular edema and reduce visual loss by >50% when used as a preventive measure to limit neovascularization and vitreous hemorrhages. Panretinal laser treatment has been proven effective and is the treatment of choice for patients with proliferative retinopathy and high-risk characteristics. A scatter pattern of 1200 to 1600 burns are applied throughout the periphery of the retina, avoiding the macular area.

Vitrectomy may be required to treat retinal detachment and large vitreous hemorrhages. This procedure generally is reserved for patients with poor vision in whom the benefits outweigh the risks.

It is also important to note that if a patient's A1C is very high (especially >10%), indicating poor control, and there is preexisting retinopathy (particularly preproliferative disease), the retinopathy can worsen if the A1C is brought down too quickly. This is especially common before pregnancy and after conception, and such patients need to have more frequent eye exams.

■ **Diabetic Nephropathy**

Over 20% of adults who have had diabetes for 20 years or more have clinically apparent nephropathy. This disease is progressive, takes years to develop, and requires laboratory evaluation for early detection because it generally is asymptomatic in the early stages.

Structural and functional changes in the kidneys occur early in the course of poorly controlled diabetes but do not produce clinical symptoms. The first sign of nephropathy is microalbuminuria (albumin excretion 30 to 300 mg/24 hours). In addition, hyperfiltration, indicated by an elevated creatinine clearance, is also a finding in early diabetic nephropathy. The important clinical point is that in this early stage of nephropathy, aggressive management may reverse or completely stabilize any abnormalities. Overt nephropathy is defined as urinary protein excretion >0.5 g/24 hours and clinical proteinuria characterized by albumin excretion rates >300 mg (0.3 g)/24 hours, typically accompanied by hypertension. The following conditions play a role in the development and acceleration of renal insufficiency:

- Chronic uncontrolled hyperglycemia
- Hypertension (virtually all patients who develop nephropathy also have hypertension [systolic blood pressure >135 mm Hg, diastolic blood pressure >85 mm Hg])
- Neurogenic bladder leading to hydronephrosis and infections
- Urinary tract infection (UTI) and obstruction
- Nephrotoxic drugs (nonsteroidal anti-inflammatory drugs, chronic analgesic abuse, radiocontrast dyes [should be used only when adequate hydration and diuresis can be assured and if no other diagnostic alternatives are available]).

14

Patients with diabetes often develop uremia at lower creatinine levels than patients with renal insufficiency resulting from other causes. Second, even with dialysis, the prognosis for patients with diabetes is worse than that for nondiabetic patients. Patients with diabetes tend to start dialysis earlier because they develop symptoms sooner than other patients with renal disease. Therefore, a renal transplant is the preferred method of treatment, if possible, at this stage.

Screening

According to current recommendations, screening for proteinuria should be done yearly, starting 5 years after puberty or from the time of diagnosis of type 1 diabetes (**Figure 14.4**). Initial screen for nephropathy can occur with a standard urine dipstick for proteinuria. A positive reading will detect approximately 500 mg/day proteinuria, which is equivalent to approximately 300 mg/day albuminuria, the hallmark of diabetic nephropathy, reflecting both histologic and functional abnormality of the kidneys. This "dipstick-positive" proteinuria is also termed clinical nephropathy, gross proteinuria, and macroproteinuria. If dipstick-positive proteinuria is detected, further screening for a milder degree of nephropathy (microalbuminuria, defined as 30 to 300 mg/day albuminuria) is not required. Rather, with this more advanced amount of proteinuria, quantification with a 24-hour urine collection for total proteinuria and creatinine clearance should be performed. Treatment should proceed accordingly (see following *Treatment* section). If the dipstick for proteinuria is negative, screening for microalbuminuria should be performed.

There are a number of methods used for screening for microalbuminuria, including a spot albumin-to-creatinine ratio, a dipstick that measures for microalbuminuria, a timed urine collection for albuminuria (eg, 4 or 8 hours), and a 24-hour urine collection. If the finding is negative, current recommendations call for repeating the measurement in 1 year. If it is positive, it needs to be repeated and shown to be positive before the diagnosis of microalbuminuria can be confirmed because numerous false-positives can occur (**Table 14.1**). To diagnose microalbuminuria, two of the three screening tests need to be positive. The 24-hour urine collection

FIGURE 14.4 — Algorithm for Screening for Diabetic Nephropathy

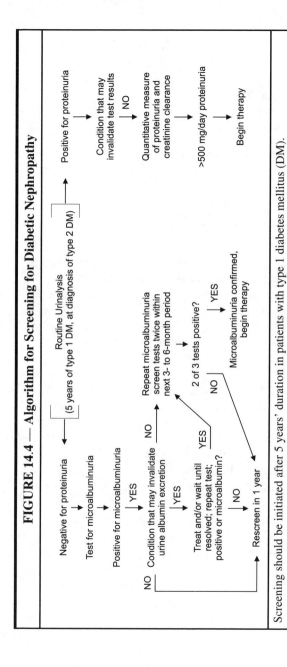

Screening should be initiated after 5 years' duration in patients with type 1 diabetes mellitus (DM).

Hirsch IB, Trence DL, eds. *Optimizing Diabetes Care for the Practitioner.* Philadelphia, Pa: Lippincott Williams and Wilkins; 2003.

14

TABLE 14.1 — Etiologies of False-Positive Tests for Microalbuminuria

- Uncontrolled hyperglycemia
- Uncontrolled hypertension
- Menstrual bleeding
- Urinary tract infection
- Exercise just prior to or during collection
- High-protein diet just prior to collection
- Thyrotoxicosis

Hirsch IB, Trence DL, eds. *Optimizing Diabetes Care for the Practitioner*. Philadelphia, Pa: Lippincott Williams and Wilkins; 2003:72.

has a better sensitivity than the other methods, and many clinicians prefer to confirm microalbuminuria with this more sensitive, albeit inconvenient, test.

It is important for physicians to inform patients with diabetes about the relationship between high blood pressure and renal disease, and the benefits of maintaining glycemic control. Patients should be encouraged to:

- Have their blood pressure checked regularly (in addition to obtaining their own blood pressure cuff to measure blood pressure at home) and take antihypertensive medications that have been prescribed
- Decrease their protein intake to approximately 10% of daily calories
- Monitor glucose levels frequently with self-monitoring of blood glucose (SMBG) and take any other measures to improve glycemia.

The importance of reporting symptoms of UTI should be emphasized, along with following proper treatment for this infection and avoiding nephrotoxic drugs.

Treatment

Treatment is aimed at early detection and prevention, focusing specifically on improving glycemic control, aggressively treating hypertension (eg, with angiotensin-converting enzyme [ACE] inhibitor or angiotensin-receptor blocker [ARB] therapy and other agents as necessary), and restricting protein intake. If proteinuria is persistent or progressive, hypertension does not respond to treatment, or serum creatinine continues to be elevated, a nephrologist should be consulted. There is also evidence that treating an elevated LDL cholesterol level and taking antioxidants such as vitamins E and C may be beneficial to the diabetic kidney, although randomized controlled trials are lacking.

Improving Glycemic Control

Considerable evidence supports the importance of optimizing glycemic control in delaying the development and slowing the progression of diabetic nephropathy. In the DCCT and the UKPDS, intensive metabolic control was associated with a decrease in the development of microalbuminuria and clinical grade proteinuria in patients with type 1 and type 2 diabetes. The benefits of improved glycemia appear to be greatest before the onset of macroalbuminuria; once overt diabetic nephropathy has developed, improved glycemia has little beneficial effect on the progression of renal disease.

Research has revealed a glycemic threshold for developing microalbuminuria, establishing an A1C level of <7% (normal is 4% to 6%) as the new glycemic goal, whereas previously it was <8%. The risk of developing microalbuminuria is substantially reduced at 7%.

Treating Hypertension

Controlling hypertension through aggressive therapeutic intervention can reduce proteinuria and considerably delay the progression of renal insufficiency. ACE inhibitors and ARBs offer effective anti-hypertensive effects in addition to significant delaying of the progression of diabetic nephropathy to end-stage renal disease. ACE inhibitors and ARBs decrease proteinuria by minimizing efferent glomerular vasoconstriction and reducing glomerular hyperfiltration. In cases where the glomerular filtration rate has already declined, ACE inhibitors also can partially reverse or prevent a further decrease. Recently, The Antihypertensive and Lipid-Lowering Treatment to Prevent Heart Attack Trial (ALLHAT) concluded that thiazide-type diuretics are superior to ACE inhibitors and calcium channel blockers in preventing one or more major forms of CV disease in patients with hypertension and diabetes. However, most of the patients with diabetes in the study had type 2 diabetes, and therefore it may be difficult to extrapolate these results to patients with type 1 diabetes, who are more prone to microvascular disease. Until more data become available, ACE inhibitors and ARBs should still be considered as first-line therapy in all normotensive and hypertensive patients with type 1 diabetes who have microalbuminuria or macroalbuminuria. ARBs (losartan, valsartan, irbesartan, candesartan) do not cause cough.

When blood pressure cannot be adequately controlled with the maximum dose of an ACE inhibitor or ARB, additional antihypertensive medications may be needed, such as calcium channel blockers, the diuretic hydrochlorothiazide (HCTZ), or centrally acting agents (eg, a clonidine patch). Patients with renal insufficiency and hypertension may be given a diuretic as part of the antihypertensive regimen because of related sodium and fluid retention; a loop diuretic usually is necessary if the creatinine level exceeds 2 mg/dL.

Restricting Protein Intake

Protein intake should be limited to 0.8 g/kg/day or approximately 10% of daily calories, derived primarily from lean animal and vegetable or plant sources, in patients with diabetes and evidence of nephropathy. Vegetable proteins appear to have beneficial renal effects compared with animal sources and provide an important protein supplement or substitute in low-protein diets. The value of restricting protein intake in the absence of diabetic renal disease has not been clearly demonstrated. Low-protein diets can be made more palatable with a greater variety of vegetable protein sources and increased consumption of high-fiber complex carbohydrates and monounsaturated fats.

■ Diabetic Neuropathy

The various diabetic neuropathies are one of the more common yet distressing long-term complications of diabetes, affecting 60% to 70% of patients with type 1 and type 2 diabetes. The categories of diabetic neuropathy are shown in **Table 14.2**.

Symmetric Distal Neuropathies

These neuropathies develop most often in the lower extremities, causing numbness and tingling

TABLE 14.2 — Types of Diabetic Neuropathies
Sensorimotor Peripheral Neuropathies   • Symmetric, distal, bilateral of upper/lower extremities   • Mononeuropathies   • Diabetic amyotrophy
Autonomic Neuropathies   • Gastroparesis diabeticorum   • Diabetic diarrhea   • Neurogenic bladder   • Impaired cardiovascular reflex responses   • Impotence

14

(pins-and-needles paresthesias) usually during the night. Some patients develop painful burning and stabbing symptoms that can interfere with their quality of life and may be associated with neuropathic cachexia syndrome that includes anorexia, depression, and weight loss. Treatments that have varying degrees of effectiveness, particularly for painful neuropathies, include gabapentin (Neurontin), tricyclic antidepressants, carbamazepine, phenytoin, tramadol (Ultram), and counterirritants (eg, topical capsaicin). Generally, gabapentin is the treatment of choice due to its superior side effect profile. Aspirin or propoxyphene should be prescribed as necessary for pain; narcotic analgesics generally should be avoided because of the risk of addiction with chronic use, however, in some cases, these drugs are necessary.

The antiseizure medication topiramate (Topamax) is another drug gaining recognition in the treatment of neuropathic pain syndromes. Although its exact mechanism of action is unknown, studies suggest that topiramate:

- Decreases nerve-cell excitation by blocking certain neurotransmitters from binding to glutamate receptors in the brain
- Enhances the activity of gamma-aminobutyric acid (GABA), a neurotransmitter that inhibits nerve-cell excitation in the brain
- Blocks sodium channels, thus reducing excessive nerve-cell firing.

Topiramate is typically well tolerated, but if the dose is titrated too quickly, side effects such as agitation, anxiety, nervousness, and word-finding difficulties become more pronounced. The patient should be maintained on the lowest dose possible to control symptoms.

In general, treatment strategies for painful peripheral neuropathy include initial use of nonsteroidal anti-inflammatory drugs, such as aspirin and acetaminophen (Tylenol), which can offer pain relief, especially in patients with musculoskeletal or joint abnormalities secondary to long-standing neuropathy. Gabapentin and the tricyclic antidepressants (eg, amitriptyline) remain the most commonly used drugs in the treatment of painful neuropathy. Topical capsaicin cream may be added to the patient's therapeutic regimen if neuropathic pain persists in spite of treatment with maximally tolerated doses of oral medication.

If neuropathic pain persists despite the outlined treatment regimen, referral to a specialist, for a transcutaneous electrical nerve stimulation (TENS) unit, acupuncture, or a series of local nerve blocks may be helpful, although the prognosis for pain relief in these patients is poor. A treatment flowchart for managing painful diabetic neuropathy is shown in **Figure 14.5**.

Mononeuropathy

These neuropathies can occur in virtually any cranial or peripheral nerve, are asymmetric, and have an abrupt onset. Cranial mononeuropathies are the most common, particularly involving cranial nerves III and VI, causing extraocular muscle motor paralysis and peripheral palsies. Patients can develop palsies involving the peroneal (footdrop), median, and ulnar nerves. Spontaneous recovery over 3 to 6 months is typical. Patients with diabetes are more prone to developing compression neuropathies such as carpal tunnel syndrome.

Gastroparesis

This neuropathy should be suspected in patients with nausea, vomiting, early satiety, abdominal distention, and bloating following a meal, and is secondary to delayed emptying and retention of gastric contents. The delay in gastric emptying usually is asymptomatic, although glycemic control can be affected. Postprandial hypoglycemia and delayed hyperglycemia develop

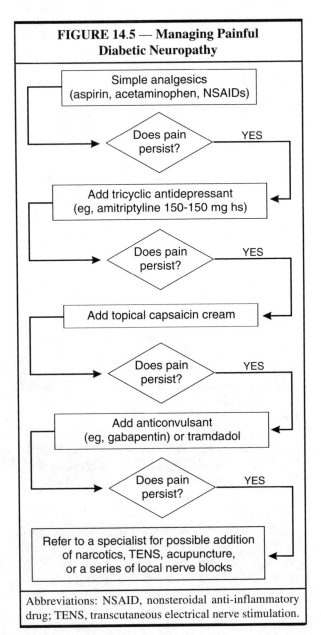

FIGURE 14.5 — Managing Painful Diabetic Neuropathy

Simple analgesics (aspirin, acetaminophen, NSAIDs)

Does pain persist? — YES

Add tricyclic antidepressant (eg, amitriptyline 150-150 mg hs)

Does pain persist? — YES

Add topical capsaicin cream

Does pain persist? — YES

Add anticonvulsant (eg, gabapentin) or tramdadol

Does pain persist? — YES

Refer to a specialist for possible addition of narcotics, TENS, acupuncture, or a series of local nerve blocks

Abbreviations: NSAID, nonsteroidal anti-inflammatory drug; TENS, transcutaneous electrical nerve stimulation.

when the balance between exogenous insulin administration and nutrient absorption is disrupted because of gastric stasis. Therefore, gastroparesis should be considered even in the absence of gastrointestinal symptoms in a patient who suddenly develops unexplained poor glycemic control after having had satisfactory control.

Primary treatment is focused on optimizing glucose control with insulin; secondary treatment involves dietary modifications in the form of low-fat, low-residue diet. When patients remain symptomatic despite these measures, treatment with the following prokinetic agents is recommended:

- Erythromycin lactobionate 1.5 to 3.0 mg/kg body weight IV every 6 to 8 hours (acute treatment, effective in eliminating residue from stomach); common side effects are nausea and vomiting.
- Oral treatment with cisapride (only obtained by special request because of cardiac side effects), 10 to 20 mg before meals and at bedtime (enhances gastric emptying through serotoninergic mechanisms, effective in acute conditions); minimal side effects (abdominal cramping, frequent bowel movements); long-term use may cause hyperprolactinemia, galactorrhea, and menstrual irregularities. The Food and Drug Administration (FDA) has placed severe restrictions on the use of cisapride because of the potential for cardiac dysrhythmias due to prolongation of the QT interval, especially when the medication is taken with agents that delay the metabolism of cisapride, such as erythromycin, clarithromycin, fluconazole, idinavir, and other agents that inhibit the cytochrome P34A system. Currently, cisapride is available only through the FDA directly and only for patients

14

in whom other therapies have failed and who meet strict criteria for the drug.

- Oral metoclopramide HCl is generally used with caution because of adverse reactions (nervousness, anxiety, dystonic effects, and the potential for irreversible tardive dyskinesia). For women, menstrual irregularity and galactorrhea due to elevated prolactin levels are common side effects. Outpatient use of subcutaneous (SC) metoclopramide is more effective than oral use for some patients.
- Oral treatment with domperidone, a peripheral dopamine antagonist (available in Canada, but not the United States), 10 to 20 mg 3 to 4 times daily (accelerates gastric emptying); minimal side effects (abdominal cramping, frequent bowel movements) and rare adverse reactions (hyperprolactinemia, galactorrhea)
- Tegaserod (Zelnorm), a $5\text{-}HT_4$-receptor agonist, has been shown to be effective for the short-term treatment of women with constipation-predominant irritable bowel syndrome. The dosage is 6 mg taken twice daily orally before meals for 4 to 6 weeks.

Diabetic Diarrhea

Intermittent diarrhea may alternate with constipation and can be difficult to treat. Diabetic diarrhea is a diagnosis of exclusion. High-fiber intake can be helpful, along with diphenoxylate (Lomotil), loperamide (Imodium), or clonidine. Small-intestine stasis contributes to bacterial overgrowth, causing diarrhea. Treatment with one of the following antibiotics for 10 to 14 days is recommended:

- Doxycycline hyclate, 100 mg every 12 hours
- Amoxicillin trihydrate, 250 mg every 6 hours
- Metronidazole, 250 mg every 6 hours
- Ciprofloxacin HCl, 250 mg every 12 hours.

A trial of pancreatic enzymes is also recommended to rule out exocrine pancreatic insufficiency. In many instances, tincture of opium is the only medication that can help the patient live a nearly normal daily life. When diarrhea does not respond to these measures, the use of SC octreotide works well.

Neurogenic Bladder

Frequent small voidings and incontinence that may progress to urinary retention characterize this neuropathy. Confirmation of this diagnosis requires demonstration of cystometric abnormalities and large residual urine volume. Most medical treatment is inadequate, although scheduling frequent voidings every 3 to 4 hours combined with bethanechol 10 to 50 mg 3 to 4 times daily supplemented by small doses of phenoxybenzamine may be helpful. Surgical intervention may be necessary if patients do not respond to pharmacologic therapy because chronic urinary retention can lead to UTI. Also, self-catheterization can be used for those in whom distention and frequent infection occur.

Impaired Cardiovascular Reflexes

Orthostatic hypotension and fixed tachycardia are the most disturbing and disabling autonomic symptoms. Typical treatment of orthostatic hypotension includes elevating the head of the bed, compression stockings for lower limbs and torso, supplementary salt intake, and the use of fludrocortisone (0.05 mg initially with gradual increases of 0.1 mg up to 0.5 to 1 mg). This pharmacologic therapy should be used cautiously in patients with cardiac disease because it causes sodium and water retention and may precipitate congestive heart failure (CHF).

14

Sexual Dysfunction

Erectile dysfunction, or impotence, is an under-recognized, underdiscussed, and commonly untreated complication of diabetes. However, it is also one of the more treatable diabetic complications. It is a couple's disorder, as both patient and partner suffer. Diabetic impotence is usually caused by circulatory and nervous system abnormalities. The classic clinical picture includes a patient with normal sexual desire but the inability to physically act on that desire. If a patient says that he has morning erections, he can masturbate without problems, or his libido is abnormally low, look for other causes of impotence such as psychological problems or a low androgen state. Orgasm and ejaculation are usually normal. Even if the patient does not have any psychological problems that could cause the impotence, he may develop a secondary psychological fear of failure that could complicate the clinical picture. A woman may experience lack of lubrication and painful intercourse.

The diagnosis can be made in most cases by a good sexual, psychosocial, and medical history, a physical examination, and laboratory tests. A testosterone level should be obtained to rule out a low androgen state, which is rarely a cause of impotence.

Hyperprolactinemia is also an uncommon cause of impotence. Hemochromatosis is a condition that is underdiagnosed and is associated with impotence and glucose intolerance. Serum iron stores, including ferritin levels, are abnormally high in this disorder. If the patient has femoral bruits and/or peripheral occlusive disease, a vascular workup may help identify the cause of impotence.

It is important to be sure the patient is not taking any medications that can cause impotence such as β-blockers and thiazide diuretics. ACE inhibitors, ARBs, calcium channel blockers, and α-blockers do not generally cause impotence.

There are now three oral medications available in the United States for the treatment of erectile dysfunction:

- Sildenafil (Viagra)
- Vardenafil (Levitra)
- Tadalafil (Cialis).

These drugs, known as selective inhibitors of phosphodiesterase type 5 (PDE5), work by inhibiting cyclic guanosine monophosphate (cGMP)-specific PDE5, resulting in smooth muscle relaxation and inflow of blood into the penile tissue upon sexual stimulation. They have become the treatment of choice for most men with erectile dysfunction. Sildenafil takes effect in about 30 minutes and the effects last approximately 4 hours; vardenafil is faster acting, reaching maximum concentration in 30 to 40 minutes; tadalafil reaches maximum concentration in 24 hours, the effects last approximately 3 days.

The recommended dose of sildenafil is 25 mg, 50 mg, or 100 mg 1 hour before sexual activity. Following an initial starting dose of 50 mg, the dose may be increased or decreased based on efficacy and tolerability. Maximum dose is 100 mg. Side effects of the medication are headaches, light-headedness, dizziness, flushing, distorted vision, dyspepsia, syncope, and myocardial infarction (MI). Men at highest risk for syncope are those taking nitrates. It also has adverse effects in people with hypertrophic cardiomyopathy because of a decrease in preload and afterload, which can increase the outflow obstruction, culminating in an unstable hemodynamic state. The American College of Cardiology and the American Heart Association have published recommendations for the use of sildenafil. The document reiterates caution with respect to the use of sildenafil in the following situations:

- Patients with active coronary ischemia who are not taking nitrates

14

- CHF and borderline blood pressure or low volume status
- Complicated, multidrug, antihypertensive regimen
- Patients taking drugs that prolong the half-life by blocking enzyme CYP3A4 (ie, erythromycin, cimetidine).

For vardenafil, the recommended dose is 10 mg taken 1 hour before sexual activity. A higher dose of 20 mg is available for patients whose response to the 10-mg dose is not adequate. Two lower doses (2.5 mg and 5.0 mg) are also available and may be necessary for patients taking other medicines or who have medical conditions that may decrease the body's ability to metabolize vardenafil. The drug should not be taken more than once per day. It should not be used with nitrates or with α-blockers. Patients who are allergic to sildenafil and vardenafil or who have severe cardiac disease in which sexual function is prohibited or who have the eye disease retinitis pigmentosa should strictly avoid vardenafil.

The recommended dose of tadalafil, the newest of the PDE5 inhibitors, is 20 mg taken prior to anticipated sexual activity. The maximum recommended dosing frequency is once per day. It may be taken between 30 minutes and 36 hours prior to anticipated sexual activity. Patients may initiate sexual activity at varying time points relative to dosing in order to determine their own optimal window of responsiveness. The dose may be lowered to 10 mg based on individual response and tolerability. Side effects of tadalafil are similar to those of the other PDE5 inhibitors and, as with the others, tadalafil should be avoided in patients using any form of organic nitrate.

Before the advent of the PDE5 inhibitors, patients used vacuum constrictor devices, intracavernosal injection of vasoactive agents, and penile prostheses, among other cumbersome measures, for the treatment of impotence. However, these approaches have largely been supplanted by use of the oral agents described here.

Macrovascular Complications

The incidence of the three major macrovascular diseases (coronary artery, cerebrovascular, and peripheral vascular) is greater in individuals with diabetes than in nondiabetic individuals, accounting for up to 80% mortality in adults with diabetes. Currently, there is no consensus about when aggressive preventive steps are warranted to prevent coronary heart disease (CHD) in patients with type 1 diabetes. In patients without diabetes, men age >45 years and women age >55 years are deemed to be at increased risk for CHD. Certainly, preventive therapies beyond good glycemic control should be initiated in patients with type 1 diabetes even before these age thresholds. Patients should be systematically assessed for risk factors, such as hypertension, cigarette smoking, and lipid abnormalities. Additionally, even mild microalbuminuria becomes a potent risk factor for CHD and stroke events when proteinuria reaches the level of early diabetic nephropathy (300 to 1,000 mg/24 hours). At this point, lipid levels may begin to take on a more atherogenic profile, including lower high-density lipoprotein (HDL) cholesterol, increased triglyceride levels, and a trend toward larger numbers of smaller, denser LDL particles without accompanying elevations of LDL cholesterol levels.

Weight control and exercise are safe and effective methods for modifying macrovascular risk and should form the basis to which all other treatments are added. The following treatments for hypertension and dyslipidemia should be applied where appropriate.

243

■ Hypertension

Hypertension should be treated vigorously in all patients with diabetes to limit and/or prevent the development and progression of atherosclerosis, nephropathy, and retinopathy. Lowering elevated blood pressure is the most important and immediate consideration, with a therapeutic goal of <130/80 mm Hg if there is no evidence of protein in the urine. The goal for patients with isolated systolic hypertension (180 mm Hg) is 160 mm Hg; further reductions to 140 mm Hg are suggested if the treatment is well tolerated. The goal for patients with renal insufficiency should be <120/80 mm Hg.

Treatment should be initiated with a no-added–salt diet and weight loss, if necessary, with appropriate aerobic exercise. Because patients with diabetes can be uniquely affected by certain side effects of antihypertensives, physicians must be familiar with the potential complications of the classes of hypertensive drugs. One or more antihypertensive medications may be necessary to achieve satisfactory blood pressure control, and adding a second drug to small or moderate doses of the first drug often results in better control with fewer side effects than using full doses of the first agent. For more information, refer to The Seventh Report of the Joint National Committee on Prevention, Detection, Evaluation, and Treatment of High Blood Pressure (*JAMA*. 2003;289:2560-2572).

Angiotensin-Converting Enzyme Inhibitors

Angiotensin-converting enzyme inhibitors and now the ARBs commonly are the first choices for therapy because they are effective and have a low incidence of side effects. They are useful in diabetic patients with and without nephropathy. They have no negative impact on carbohydrate or lipid metabolism, can slow the rate of progression of proteinuria in diabetic nephropathy, reduce the decline in renal function,

244

and prevent progression of retinopathy. Caution should be used in patients with peripheral occlusive disease because renal artery stenosis may be present, which could lead to renal decline with ACE inhibitors.

ACE inhibitors have now been shown to be cardioprotective in addition to their beneficial effects on the diabetic kidney. The Health Outcomes Prevention Evaluation (HOPE) trial studied over 3,500 subjects with type 2 diabetes who had documentation of previous CV events and were over 55 years of age. Subjects were randomized to either ramipril (10 mg/day) or placebo and vitamin E or placebo. Within 4.5 years, the ramipril-treated group experienced a 22% reduction in MI, a 33% reduction in stroke, a 37% reduction in any CV event, and a 24% reduction in the development of overt nephropathy when compared with the placebo groups. These benefits occurred despite minor reductions in blood pressure, raising the possibility that ACE inhibitors have benefits for diabetic patients independent of blood pressure lowering. Moreover, this is consistent with the results of a smaller study focusing on patients with type 1 diabetes (n = 409) in which the authors concluded that treatment with the ACE inhibitor captopril was associated with a 50% reduction in the risk of death, dialysis, and transplantation despite modest disparities in blood pressure between the treatment and control groups. In summary, the HOPE study is a landmark study confirming the results of multiple smaller and less-powered studies demonstrating the cardiac and renal protective effects of ACE inhibitors in subjects with diabetes. Based on the results of these studies, ACE inhibitors should be considered first-line therapy in all diabetic patients with mild to moderate hypertension and/or microalbuminuria or macroalbuminuria.

Serum potassium should be monitored during therapy with ACE inhibitors in patients with suspected hyporeninemic hypoaldosteronism (type IV renal tubular acidosis) to prevent severe hyperkalemia.

Angiotensin II Receptor Blockers

Like the ACE inhibitors, ARBs have been shown to slow the progression of albuminuria and be protective in diabetic nephropathy, although almost all of the data pertain to type 2 diabetes. Empiric evidence suggests, however, that ARBs may be equally as effective in patients with type 1 diabetes. There is some evidence from the Candesartan and Lisinopril Microalbuminuria (CALM) study that combining an ACE inhibitor and an ARB reduces blood pressure and urinary albumin levels more than either agent alone.

β-Blockers

β-Blockers have been shown to be useful in treating the hypertensive patient with diabetes. Nevertheless, these agents inhibit hepatic glucose production, which may lead to hypoglycemia by masking many of its warning symptoms. β-Blockers also increase the potential for developing hyperkalemia by inhibiting resin synthesis and reducing potassium uptake by extrarenal tissues. They can also exacerbate dyslipidemia. In patients with difficult-to-control hypertension, especially with autonomic neuropathy (parasympathetic dysfunction) and tachycardia, the use of specific β_1-antagonists is preferred because they are less likely to cause hypoglycemia and hyperkalemia.

Calcium Channel Blockers

There are three subclasses of calcium channel blocker: the dihydropyridine group (dihydropyridine calcium channel blockers [DCCBs]) and the benzothiazepines and phenylalkylamines (nondihydropyridine calcium channel blockers [NDCCBs]). The DCCBs are a heterogenous class of compounds with significant pharmacologic differences and primary vasodilatory effect. Due to conflicting evidence, it is unclear whether the DCCBs reduce CV events or progression of nephropathy. They may protect against stroke, but appear to be less effective than ACE inhibitors in reducing CV events. An increase in CV mortality has been reported with the short-acting DCCB nifedipine. Short-acting DCCBs are not approved for treatment of hypertension in diabetic patients and should not be used in this population.

Use of the NDCCBs has been associated with decreased proteinuria in short-term studies of patients with overt diabetic nephropathy.

Diuretics

Low-dose thiazide diuretic use has been associated with reduced risk of CHF and stroke in large randomized trials. As discussed earlier, treatment of systolic hypertension in older diabetic subjects with low-dose thiazides significantly reduced CV events. Their effects on progression of renal impairment have not been studied in large randomized clinical trials. Low-dose thiazides probably do not impair insulin sensitivity or worsen the lipid profile as high doses have been reported to do. Low-dose thiazide diuretics may be particularly useful in combination with other antihypertensive agents. The loop diuretics have been used in combination therapy, particularly in diabetic patients with decreased renal function.

14

■ Dyslipidemia

Dyslipidemia in patients with diabetes may result from a wide variety of factors including:
- Poor metabolic control
- Use of certain drugs, such as high-dose β-blockers (excluding carvedilol), high-dose diuretics, androgens, progestins (other than micronized progesterone or despironone), estrogens, systemic corticosteroids, or protease-inhibitor antiviral agents

- Obesity
- Genetic predisposition
- Associated conditions such as hypothyroidism.

Although prevalence of dyslipidemia is no greater in patients with type 1 diabetes compared to those without, the high absolute risk of heart attack in people with type 1 diabetes warrants careful adherence to the lipid treatment guidelines discussed below.

All patients with type 1 diabetes should be screened for lipid abnormalities in the initial evaluation using a fasting lipid profile to determine serum triglyceride, total cholesterol, HDL cholesterol, and LDL cholesterol levels. Shown in **Table 14.3** are acceptable, borderline, and high-risk lipid levels for adult.

Because lipid abnormalities often reflect poor glycemic control, the first treatment approach to dyslipidemia should be optimizing diabetes management with diet, exercise, and pharmacologic therapy, as needed. As glycemic control improves, lipid levels also usually improve. Limiting calories and saturated fat intake has proved to be highly effective in improving, but not normalizing, dyslipidemia. Increased intake of soluble fiber, particularly from oat and bean products, has been shown to reduce LDL cholesterol levels. The National Cholesterol Education Program has designed a stepped approach for restricting dietary fat and cholesterol that can be modified to incorporate specific requirements for diabetic nutrition. The following guidelines should be implemented with the assistance of a registered dietitian:

- *Step 1 diet guidelines*: limit saturated fat intake to 8% to 10% of daily calories, with 30% of calories from total fat; limit cholesterol intake to <300 mg/day. If this approach is not adequate for meeting lipid goals, initiate Step 2.

TABLE 14.3 — Lipid Levels for Adults

Risk for Adult Diabetic Patients	Cholesterol	HDL Cholesterol* (mg/dL)	LDL Cholesterol (mg/dL)	Triglycerides (mg/dL)
Low	<200	>45	<100	<200
Borderline	200-239	35-45	100-129	200-399
High	≥240	<35	≥130	≥400

* For women, the HDL cholesterol values should be increased by 10 mg/dL.

American Diabetes Association. *Diabetes Care.* 2005;28(suppl 1):S4-S36.

14

- *Step 2 diet guidelines*: limit saturated fat intake to <7% of daily calories; limit cholesterol intake to <200 mg/day.
- If triglycerides are >1000 mg/dL, all dietary fats should be reduced to lower circulating chylomicrons.

Recommendations for effective diet therapy for the treatment of lipid disorders in diabetes are shown in **Table 14.4**.

The ADA follows an order of priority for the treatment of diabetic dyslipidemia. Lowering of LDL cholesterol is considered the first priority, followed by HDL cholesterol raising, triglyceride lowering, and treatment of combined hyperlipidemia. However, patients with type 1 diabetes who maintain good glycemic control tend to have normal levels of lipoproteins unless they are overweight or obese. Because observational and clinical trial data on the relationship between lipoproteins and cardiovascular disease are sparse, it is important to follow the recent ADA recommendation that all people with diabetes >40 years of age with a total cholesterol of ≥135 mg/dL should receive statin therapy,

---

TABLE 14.4 — Diet Recommendations for the Treatment of Lipid Disorders in Diabetes

- Calorie restriction and increased physical activity for weight loss as indicated
- Saturated and transunsaturated fat intake <10% and preferably <7% of total energy intake
- Total dietary cholesterol intake <200 mg/day
- Emphasis on complex carbohydrates (at least five portions per day of fruits/vegetables); soluble fibers (legumes, oats, certain fruits/vegetables) have additional benefits on total cholesterol, LDL cholesterol level, and glycemic control
- Replacing saturated fat with carbohydrate or monounsaturated fats (eg, canola oil, olive oil)

---

with the aim of reducing LDL by approximately 30% regardless of baseline LDL levels.

Diabetic Foot Disorders

More than half of all nontraumatic amputations in the United States occur in individuals with diabetes, and the majority of these could have been prevented with proper foot care. Efforts aimed at prevention, early detection, and treatment of diabetic foot disorders can have a significant impact on the incidence of these problems.

■ Detection and Treatment

The physician and patient must diligently examine the feet on a regular basis for signs of redness or trauma, especially if neuropathy is present. Lack of pain, position, and vibratory sensations caused by neuropathy, associated deformities, and vascular ischemia can facilitate the development of foot lesions. Foot pressure that is abnormally distributed predisposes a neuropathic patient to pressure ischemia and skin breakdown. Autonomic neuropathy causes decreased sweating and dry skin that can result in cracked, thickened skin that is susceptible to infection and ulceration.

Pressure perception can be assessed using the Semmes Weinstein (SW) monofilaments, which are available in three thicknesses: 1-g fiber (SW 4.17 rating), 10-g fiber (SW 5.07 rating), and 75-g fiber (SW 6.10 rating). The following evaluation procedure has been recommended:

14

Place the monofilament against the skin and apply pressure to different areas of the bottom of the foot until the filament buckles. The patient should be able to feel the monofilament when it buckles and identify the location being tested. The SW 5.07 monofilament, which is equivalent to 10 g of linear pressure, detects the presence or absence of protective sensation and is useful for identifying a foot at risk for ulceration and in need of special care.

Daily inspection of feet can help detect early skin lesions, and proper footwear can minimize the development of foot problems. Patients should be taught to cut toenails straight across and not trim calluses themselves, regularly wash their feet with warm water and mild soap, and avoid going barefoot or wearing constricting shoes. Minor wounds that are not infected can be treated with mild antiseptic solution, daily dressing changes, and foot rest. Patient guidelines for care of the diabetic foot are shown in **Table 14.5**.

Podiatrists should be consulted for assistance with more serious foot problems and for regular nail and callus care in high-risk individuals. If an ulcer develops, the skin must be débrided and the pressure alleviated; infections should be treated promptly with medications appropriate for the offending organism. Healing is facilitated by bed rest with foot elevation and the use of an orthopedic walking cast to relieve pressure but allow mobility. Intravenous antibiotics, surgical débridement, distal arterial revascularization, and local foot-sparing surgery may help prevent amputation in cases of seriously infected foot ulcers.

SUGGESTED READING

Abuaisha BB, Constanzi JB, Boulton AJ. Acupuncture for the treatment of chronic painful peripheral diabetic neuropathy: a long-term study. *Diabetes Res Clin Prac*. 1998;39:115-121.

American Diabetes Association. Management of dyslipidemia in adults with diabetes. *Diabetes Care*. 2004;27(suppl 1):S68-S71.

American Diabetes Association. *Diabetes 2002 Vital Statistics*. Alexandria, Va: American Diabetes Association; 2002.

TABLE 14.5 — Care of the Diabetic Foot

- Wash feet daily and dry carefully, especially between the toes (same after shower, Jacuzzi, or swimming).
- Inspect feet daily for blisters, cuts, scratches, and areas of possible infection. Look between the toes. A mirror can help with inspecting hard-to-see areas. Individuals who have trouble inspecting feet should seek the help of a family member or friend.
- If feet are cold at night, socks should be worn. Extreme care should be taken to test temperature of bath water and avoid hot pavement/concrete in the summer.
- Inspect shoes daily for foreign objects, nail points, torn linings, or other problems.
- Change socks daily, wear properly fitting socks, and avoid holes or mended socks. "THOR-LO" socks have extra padding in heel and ball of foot for better shock absorption (available in sporting goods stores).
- All shoes should be comfortable at the time of purchase; do not depend on shoes to break in. Wear them only 1 hour the first day, and only in the house. Check feet for blisters; slowly increase the wearing time.
- Do not wear sandals with thongs between the toes and never wear shoes without socks.
- Never walk barefoot, not even in the house, because of the danger of stepping on sharp objects on the floor.
- Do not use chemical agents to remove corns or calluses, and always leave cutting to a podiatrist, who should be told that the patient has diabetes.
- Toenails should be cut straight across. If there is concern about this, a podiatrist should be consulted.
- Infections from cuts, scratches, blisters, etc, can cause significant problems in diabetic patients; a podiatrist or physician should be seen when infection occurs.
- Cigarette smoking should be curtailed or avoided.

Adapted from: Goldman F, Gibbons G, Kruse-Edelmann I. Limb salvage techniques. In: *High Risk Foot in Diabetes Mellitus.* New York, NY: Churchill Livingstone; 1990.

Backonja M, Beydoun A, Edwards KR, et al. Gabapentin for the symptomatic treatment of painful neuropathy in patients with diabetes mellitus: a randomized controlled trial. *JAMA*. 1998;280: 1831-1836.

Cheitlin MD, Hutter AM Jr, Brindis RG, et al. Use of sildenafil (Viagra) in patients with cardiovascular disease. Technology and Practice Executive Committee. *Circulation*. 1999;99:168-177.

Chu NV, Edelman SV. Erectile dysfunction and diabetes. *Curr Diab Rep*. 2002;2:60-66.

Cohen KL, Harris S. Efficacy and safety of nonsteroidal anti-inflammatory drugs in the therapy of diabetic neuropathy. *Arch Intern Med*. 1987;147:1442-1444.

Collins R, Armitage J, Parish S, Sleigh P, Peto R, Heart Protection Study Collaborative Group. MRC/BHF Heart Protection Study of cholesterol-lowering with simvastatin in 5963 people with diabetes: a randomised placebo-controlled trial. *Lancet*. 2003;361: 2005-2016.

Davidson MB. *Diabetes Mellitus: Diagnosis and Treatment*. 3rd ed. New York, NY: Churchill Livingstone; 1991.

The Diabetes Control and Complications Trial Research Group. The effect of intensive treatment of diabetes on the development and progression of long-term complications in insulin-dependent diabetes mellitus. *N Engl J Med*. 1993;329:977-986.

The Diabetic Retinopathy Study Research Group. Indications for photocoagulation treatment of diabetic retinopathy, Dibetic Retinopathy Study Report No. 14. *Int Ophthalmol Clin*. 1987;27:239-253.

Early Treatment Diabetic Retinopathy Study research group. Photocoagulation for diabetic macular edema: Early Treatment Diabetic Retinopathy Study report number 1. *Arch Ophthalmol*. 1985;103:1796-1806.

Edelman SV, Henry RR. *Diagnosis and Management of Type 2 Diabetes*. 5th ed. Caddo, Okla: Professional Communications, Inc; 2002.

Goldman F, Gibbons G, Kruse-Edelmann I. Limb salavage techniques. In: *High Risk Foot in Diabetes Mellitus*. New York, NY: Churchill Livingstone; 1990.

Gorson KC, Schott C, Herman R, Ropper AH, Rand WM. Gabapentin in the treatment of painful diabetic neuropathy: a placebo controlled, double blind, crossover trial. *J Neurol Neurosurg Psychiatry*. 1999;66:251-252.

Harati Y, Gooch C, Swenson M, et al. Double-blind randomized trial of tramadol for the treatment of the pain of diabetic neuropathy. *Neurology*. 1998;50:1842-1846.

Heart Outcomes Prevention Evaluation Study Investigators. Effects of ramipril on cardiovascular and microvascular outcomes in people with diabetes mellitus: results of the HOPE study and MICRO-HOPE substudy. *Lancet*. 2000;355:253-259.

Hirsch IB, Trence DL, eds. *Optimizing Diabetes Care for the Practitioner*. Philadelphia, Pa: Lippincott Williams and Wilkins; 2003.

Karlsson FO, Garber AJ. Prevention and treatment of diabetic nephropathy: role of angiotensin-converting enzyme inhibitors. *Endocr Pract*. 1996;2:215-219.

Krolewski AS, Laffel LM, Krolewski M, Quinn M, Warram JH. Glycosylated hemoglobin and the risk of microalbuminuria in patients with insulin-dependent diabetes mellitus. *N Engl J Med*. 1995;332:1251-1255.

Kumar D, Marshall HJ. Diabetic peripheral neuropathy: amelioration of pain with transcutaneous electrostimulation. *Diabetes Care*. 1997;20:1702-1705.

Labasky RC, Spivack AP. Transurethral alprostadil for treatment of erectile dysfunction: two-year safety update. *J Urol*. 1998;159:907A.

Lakin MM, Montague DK, VanderBrug Medendorp S, Tesar L, Schover LR. Intracavernous injection therapy: analysis of results and complications. *J Urol*. 1990;143:1138-1141.

Leungwattanakij S, Flynn V Jr, Hellstrom WJ. Intracavernosal injection and intraurethral therapy for erectile dysfunction. *Urol Clin North Am*. 2001;28:343-354.

Levine LA, Dimitiou RJ. Vacuum constriction and external erection devices in erectile dysfunction. *Urol Clin North Am*. 2001;28:355-361.

14

Lewis EJ, Hunsicker LG, Bain RP, Rohde RD. The effect of angiotensin-converting–enzyme inhibition on diabetic nephropathy. The Collaborative Study Group. *N Engl J Med*. 1993;329:1456-1462.

Max MB, Culnane M, Schafer SC, et al. Amitriptyline relieves diabetic neuropathy pain in patients with normal or depressed mood. *Neurology*. 1987;37:589-596.

Mayfield JA, Reiber GE, Sanders LJ, Janisse D, Pogach LM, American Diabetes Association. Preventive foot care in people with diabetes. *Diabetes Care*. 2003;26(suppl 1):S78-S79.

McQuay HJ, Tramer M, Nye BA, Carroll D, Wiffen PJ, Moore RA. A systematic review of antidepressants in neuropathic pain. *Pain*. 1996;68:217-227.

Montague DK, Angermeier KW. Penile prosthesis implantation. *Urol Clin North Am*. 2001;28:355-361.

Mudaliar SR, Henry RR. Role of glycemic control and protein restriction in clinical management of diabetic kidney disease. *Endocrinol Pract*. 1996;2:220-226.

Padma-Nathan H, Giuliano F. Oral drug therapy for erectile dysfunction. *Urol Clin North Am*. 2001;28:321-334.

Pergallo-Dittko V, ed. *A Core Curriculum for Diabetes Education*. 2nd ed. Chicago, Ill: American Association of Diabetes Educators; 1993.

Prather CM. Evaluating and managing GI dysfunction in diabetes. *Contemp Intern Med*. 1996;8:47-54.

Reichard P, Nilsson BY, Rosenqvist U. The effect of long-term intensified insulin treatment on the development of microvascular complications of diabetes mellitus. *N Engl J Med*. 1993;329:304-309.

Rendell MS, Rajfer J, Wicker PA, Smith MD. Sildenafil for treatment of erectile dysfunction in men with diabetes: a randomized controlled trial. Sildenafil Diabetes Study Group. *JAMA*. 1999;281:421-426.

Wolosin JD, Edelman SV. Diabetes and the gastrointestinal tract. *Clin Diabetes*. 2000;18:148-151.

*Note: Entries followed by
"f" indicate figures; "t" tables.*

15

15

15

15

15

15

15

15

15

15

15

15